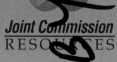

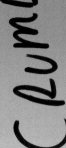

MW01505332

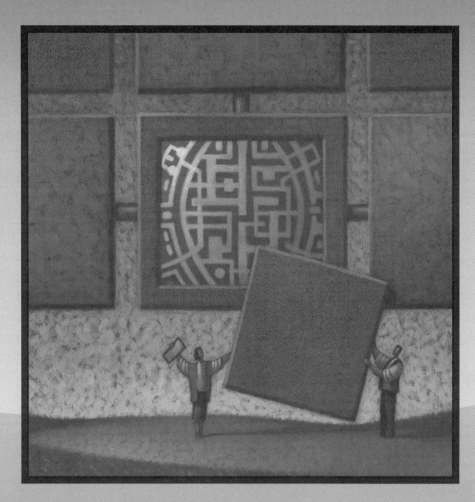

Root Cause Analysis in Health Care

Tools and Techniques

SECOND EDITION

Improving Health Care Quality and Safety

Joint Commission Resources Mission

The mission of Joint Commission Resources is to continuously improve the safety and quality of care in the United States and in the international community through the provision of education and consultation services and international accreditation.

Joint Commission Resources educational programs and publications support, but are separate from, the accreditation activities of the Joint Commission. Attendees at Joint Commission Resources educational programs and purchasers of Joint Commission Resources publications receive no special consideration or treatment in, or confidential information about, the accreditation process.

Printed in the U.S.A. 5 4 3 2 1
Requests for permission to reprint or make copies of any part of this book should be addressed to
Permissions Editor
Joint Commission Resources
One Renaissance Boulevard
Oakbrook Terrace, IL 60181

ISBN: 0-86688-781-4
Library of Congress Catalog Number: 2002110347

For more information about Joint Commission Resources, please visit our Web site at www.jcrinc.com.

This publication is designed to provide accurate and authoritative information in regard to the subject matter covered. Every attempt has been made to ensure accuracy at the time of publication; however, please note that laws, regulations, and standards are subject to change. Please also note that some of the examples in this publication are specific to the laws and regulations of the locality of the facility. The information and examples in this publication are provided with the understanding that the publisher is not engaged in providing medical, legal, or other professional advice. If any such assistance is desired, the services of a competent professional person should be sought.

Table of Contents

Introduction

Despite remarkable advances in almost every field of medicine, an age-old problem continues to haunt health care professionals—the occurrence of errors or *failures*—the term used increasingly instead of *errors*. When such failures harm individuals receiving health care services, the problem is extremely disturbing. Many, if not most, failures and sentinel events are the result of systems problems. These problems inherently cause failures to occur and individuals to be harmed. Although the rate of such failures in health care is unknown (and may be unknowable), any failure, error, or sentinel event is a cause for concern. These events can result in tragedy for individuals served and their families, add cost to an already overburdened health care system, adversely affect the public's perception of an organization, and lead to wasteful litigation. They can also deeply affect health care professionals who are dedicated to helping individuals receiving care, treatment, or service. Why do these things happen?

The Current Health Care Environment

Health care continues to experience dramatic change. As health care organizations become more complex, their systems and processes are increasingly interdependent and often interlocked or coupled. This makes the opportunity for failure more frequent and the recovery from failure by those involved more difficult. The rapid explosion of the medical knowledge base has made it increasingly challenging for practitioners to stay up to date. Yet, despite technological advances and great gains in knowledge, health care systems are, and will continue to be, appropriately dependent on human intervention. The rigorous financial constraints imposed by managed care and the need to reduce health care expenditures have affected every type of health care organization. No organization is immune. Organization leaders are reassessing their workforces. Workloads are heavier, creating increased stress and fatigue for health care professionals. Caregivers are working in new settings and performing new functions, sometimes with minimal training. Skill mixes are shifting. In short, the health care environment is ripe for serious problems caused by systems failures.

Instances of errors and sentinel events within health care organizations have been reported in the media with increasing regularity. These events cast a shadow on the public's trust of health care. People justifiably ask, "What's going on?" A galvanized industry is responding. Failure detection, reduction, and prevention strategies are receiving needed new impetus as the health care industry recognizes the need for a proactive approach to reduce the risk of failure. Regulatory and accrediting agencies have both formulated new requirements regarding failure or sentinel event reporting and suggested strategies for prevention.

When an adverse or sentinel event occurs, organizations must develop an understanding of the root causes of the event—the fundamental reasons a problem has occurred—and the interrelationship of causes. Next, the organization must implement improvement or redesign efforts to eliminate causative factors. It is clear that general knowledge about adverse events is limited, at best. General knowledge is even more limited in the area of proactive design or redesign of health care processes and systems. These aim to prevent, or at least minimize, the likelihood of

1

future failures and to protect individuals from the effects of failures when they do occur.

Purpose of the Book

Root Cause Analysis in Health Care: Tools and Techniques, Second Edition aims to help health care organizations prevent systems failures by using root cause analysis to identify causes of a sentinel event, to implement risk reduction strategies that decrease the likelihood of a recurrence of the event, and to identify effective and efficient ways of improving performance.

Root cause analysis is an effective technique most commonly used *after* "something bad" has occurred in order to identify underlying causes. Failure mode and effects analysis (FMEA), also recommended by the Joint Commission, is a proactive technique used to prevent process and product problems *before* they occur. Health care organizations should learn both techniques in order to reduce the likelihood of adverse events. This book on root cause analysis and its companion on FMEA[1] outline both approaches in a step-by-step manner.

Root Cause Analysis in Health Care: Tools and Techniques, Second Edition provides readers with up-to-date information on the Joint Commission's Sentinel Event Policy and new safety-related requirements. It also includes new examples that guide the reader through application of root cause analysis to the investigation of specific types of sentinel events, such as a medication error,* suicide, treatment delay, and elopement. For ease of access and use by root cause analysis teams, practical checklists and worksheets are now offered at the end of each chapter.

This publication provides and explains the Joint Commission's framework for conducting a root cause analysis. It also helps organizations to

* identify the processes that could benefit from root cause analysis;
* conduct a thorough and credible root cause analysis;
* interpret analysis results;
* develop and implement an action plan for improvement;
* assess the effectiveness of risk reduction efforts; and
* integrate root cause analysis with other programs.

It is our hope that even without the occurrence of an adverse event, health care organizations will embrace the use of root cause analysis to investigate "near misses" in order to minimize the possibility of future failures and, thereby, to improve the care, treatment, and service provided at their facilities.

Overview of Contents

Root Cause Analysis in Health Care: Tools and Techniques, Second Edition provides health care organizations with practical, "how to" information on conducting a root cause analysis. Twenty-one "steps" are described. Teams conducting a root cause analysis might not follow these steps in a sequential order. Often, numerous steps will occur simultaneously or the team will return to earlier steps before proceeding to the next step. It is critical for teams to customize or adapt the process to meet the unique needs of the team and organization. Appropriate tools for use in each stage of root cause analysis are identified in each chapter. A chapter-by-chapter look at the contents follows.

Chapter 1. Root Cause Analysis: An Overview provides an overview of root cause analysis. It describes variation and how proximate and root causes differ, when root cause analysis can be conducted, and the benefits of root cause analysis. One of the benefits involves effectively meeting new Joint Commission requirements that relate to the management of sentinel events. The chapter also provides guidelines on the characteristics of a thorough and credible root cause analysis and action plan. It outlines the minimum scope of root cause analysis for ten specific types of sentinel events required by the Joint Commission.

---

* The Joint Commission defines a *medication error* as a discrepancy between what a physician orders and what is reported to occur (adapted from the Joint Commission's *2002 Comprehensive Accreditation Manual for Hospitals: The Official Handbook*).

Chapter 2. Developing and Implementing a Policy and an Early Response Strategy for Sentinel Events describes the types of adverse events occurring in health care and the role played in risk reduction and prevention in an organization's culture and by its leadership. The Joint Commission's Sentinel Event Policy and requirements are provided in full, including a description of reportable and reviewable events. The chapter also includes practical guidelines on how an organization can develop its own sentinel event policy. It describes the need for root cause analysis and provides practical guidance on the early steps involved in responding to an adverse or sentinel event. These include prompt and appropriate care provided to the individual served, risk containment to minimize the possibility of a similar event recurring immediately with other individuals served, event investigation so that the organization can explore exactly what occurred and learn from the event, and appropriate communication and disclosure to relevant parties.

Chapter 3. Preparing for Root Cause Analysis covers the early steps involved in performing a root cause analysis. The first of four hands-on workbook chapters, it describes how to organize a root cause analysis team, define the problem, and gather the information and measurement data to study the problem. Details are provided about team composition and meeting ground rules. The chapter also covers how to use information gleaned from the Joint Commission's Sentinel Event Database and accreditation requirements to identify problem areas in need of root cause analysis. Risk points and failure-prone systems are described, as is a method for developing an aim statement for a preliminary root cause analysis plan. Finally, the chapter provides guidance on recording information obtained during a root cause analysis, interviewing techniques, and gathering physical and documentary evidence.

Chapter 4. Determining What Happened and Why: The Search for Proximate Causes provides practical guidance on the next stage of root cause analysis—

determining what happened and why. Organized in a workbook format, the chapter describes how to further define the event; identify process problems; determine which care processes are involved with the problem; and pinpoint the human, process, equipment, environmental, and other factors closest to the problem. The chapter also addresses how to collect and assess data on proximate and underlying causes. It provides guidance on choosing what to measure, describes indicators or measures, and guides teams through the process of ensuring that the data collected are appropriate to the desired measurement. In addition, the chapter describes the process of designing and implementing interim changes.

Chapter 5. Identifying Root Causes provides practical guidance, through workbook questions, on identifying or uncovering the root causes—the systems that lie underneath or behind sentinel events—and the interrelationship of the root causes to each other and other health care processes. Systems are explored and described, including human resources, information management, environment of care, leadership, communication, and uncontrollable factors. The chapter also addresses how to differentiate root causes and contributing causes. The most frequently occurring root causes identified by organizations that experienced a medication-related sentinel event, a restraint-related death, suicide in a 24-hour care setting, and wrong-site surgery are provided.

Chapter 6. Designing and Implementing an Action Plan for Improvement includes practical guidelines on how to design and implement an action plan—the improvement portion of a root cause analysis. During this stage, an organization identifies risk reduction strategies and designs and implements improvement strategies to address underlying systems problems. Characteristics of an acceptable action plan are provided, as is information on how to assess the effectiveness of improvement efforts. The chapter concludes with information on how to communicate the results in improvement initiatives.

Chapter 7. Tools and Techniques presents the tools and techniques used during root cause analysis. Each tool "profile" addresses the purpose of the tool, the appropriate stage(s) of root cause analysis for the tool's use, simple steps for success, and tips for effective use. Tools and techniques include affinity diagrams, barrier analysis, brainstorming, cause-and-effect diagrams, change analysis, control charts, failure mode and effect analysis, fault tree analysis, flowcharts, Gantt charts, histograms, multivoting, Pareto charts, run charts, scatter diagrams, and time lines.

Chapter 8. Case Study: A Sample Infant Abduction Root Cause Analysis provides a sample root cause analysis conducted by an organization that experienced an infant abduction. The story of a real-life incident at one hospital is shared, and the tools and techniques used to dig down to the root causes of the event are identified and explained.

Finally, the *Glossary of Terms* provides definitions of key terms used throughout the book and the *Selected Bibliography* guides readers to pertinent information sources.

A Word About Terminology

The terms *individual served, patient*, and *care recipient* all describe the individual, client, consumer, or resident who actually receives health care, treatment, and/or service. The term *care* includes care, treatment, service, rehabilitation, habilitation, or other programs instituted by the organization for individuals served.

Acknowledgments

We wish to express sincere thanks to our primary contacts at St. Joseph's Hospital and Medical Center in Paterson, New Jersey—the organization providing the sample root cause analysis included in Chapter 8 of this publication. Our gratitude goes to Barbara A. Niedz, PhD, RN, director of quality management, and Patricia DeBernardo, RN, nurse manager. These individuals worked closely with us and invested many hours to provide the information needed to tell the infant abduction root cause analysis story in a way that would help their colleagues at other organizations.

We also would like to thank three individuals who helped to provide practical examples throughout the publication. Many thanks to Judy B. Courtemanche, RN, MS, field representative surveyor for the Joint Commission; Robin S. Diamond, MSN, JD, RN, health care consultant for Medical Assurance, Inc., Coppell, Texas; and Kate M. Fenner, PhD, partner, Compass Group, Cincinnati, Ohio. Two individuals—Janet Sonnenberg, RN, MS, and Robert Katzfey—deserve special thanks for their careful review of the first edition of this publication and for providing recommendations regarding material that should be added to the second edition. Our thanks also goes to Nancy Gorham Haiman for her outstanding job writing and revising this book.

References

1. Joint Commission Resources. *Failure Mode and Effects Analysis (FMEA): Proactive Risk Reduction*. Oakbrook Terrace, IL: JCR, 2002.

Chapter 1

Root Cause Analysis: An Overview

What Is Root Cause Analysis?

Root cause analysis is a process for identifying the basic or causal factors that underlie variation in performance. Variation in performance can (and often does) produce unexpected and undesired adverse outcomes, including the occurrence of or risk of a sentinel event. The Joint Commission defines *sentinel event* as an unexpected occurrence involving death or serious physical or psychological injury, or the risk thereof (see Chapter 2, page 21). A root cause analysis focuses primarily on systems and processes, not individual performance. To be successful, it must not assign blame. Rather, through the root cause analysis process, a team works to understand a process or processes, the causes or potential causes of variation, and process changes that would make variation less likely to occur in the future. Root cause analysis examines special causes in clinical processes and common causes in organization processes to identify potential process or system improvements.

A *root cause* is the most fundamental reason a failure, or a situation where performance does not meet expectations, has occurred. In common usage, the word *cause* suggests responsibility or a factor to blame for a problem. In this book, however, the use of the word *cause* implies no assignment of blame. Instead, the cause refers to a relationship or potential relationship between certain factors that enable a sentinel event to occur. Our focus in this publication is on a positive, preventive approach to system change following a sentinel event or "near miss" sentinel event—one which almost occurred. Root cause analysis can do more than resolve that "A caused B." The process can also help an organization determine that "if we change

A because we had a problem with it, we can reduce the possibility of B recurring or, in fact, prevent B from occurring in the first place."

When Can a Root Cause Analysis Be Performed?

Root cause analysis is most commonly used *reactively*—to probe the reason for a bad outcome or for failures that have already occurred. Root cause analysis can also be used to probe a "near miss" event or as a part of other performance improvement redesign initiatives, such as understanding variation in systematically collected data. The best root cause analyses look at the entire process and support systems involved in a specific event in order to minimize overall risk associated with that process, as well as the recurrence of the event that prompted the root cause analysis.[1] The product of the root cause analysis is an *action plan* that identifies the strategies that the organization intends to implement to reduce the risk of similar events occurring in the future.

Root cause analysis is also used increasingly by organizations as one step of a proactive risk reduction effort using failure mode and effects analysis (FMEA; see Chapter 7, or pages 153–154). FMEA is a *proactive*, prospective approach used to prevent process and product problems before they occur. It provides a look not only at what problems could occur, but at how severe the effects of those problems could be. Its goal is to prevent poor results, which in health care means "harm to individuals served." One step of FMEA involves identifying the root causes of failures or "failure modes" created by special-cause variation.[2] A root cause analysis approach is used at this point in the FMEA process.

This publication focuses on the use of root cause analysis to probe the underlying reasons for a sentinel event that has occurred or nearly occurred. In the nuclear power and aerospace industries, sentinel events are rare because they have been anticipated. Systems, often with significant redundancies, have been built to protect against them. In contrast, sentinel events in the health care environment, involving death or serious injury or the risk thereof, occur with relative frequently and tend to be handled largely in a reactive way. Research studies on the frequency of errors occurring in health care cite significant adverse event rates ranging from 3.7% to 6.5%.[3,4]

Fundamentally, sentinel events in all environments provide two challenges:

- To understand how and why the event occurred; and
- To prevent the same or a similar event from occurring in the future through prospective process design or redesign.

To meet these challenges, organizations must understand not only the *proximate causes* (the superficial, obvious, or immediate causes) of the event but, more important, the *underlying causes* (the causes that led to the proximate causes) and the interrelationship of causes. Root cause analysis helps organizations look underneath the apparent proximate causes to get at the root of a sentinel event (see Figure 1-1, page 7).

Conducting a root cause analysis has significant resource implications. A team approach, involving a full range of disciplines and departments involved in the process being studied, is mandatory, as described in Chapter 3. Organizations therefore will want to conduct root cause analysis principally to explore those events or possible events with a significant negative or potentially negative impact on care outcomes.

Variation and the Difference Between Proximate and Root Causes

Adverse or sentinel events involve unexpected variation in a process. When this variation occurs, there is a chance of a serious adverse outcome. As mentioned previously, root cause analysis is a process for identifying the basic or causal factors that underlie variation in performance. According to *Webster's, variation* is a change in the form, position, state, or qualities of a thing. Although a sentinel event is the result of an unexpected variation in a process, variation is inherent in every process. To reduce the variation, it is necessary to determine its cause. In fact, variation can be classified by cause.

Common-cause variation, although inherent in every process, is a consequence of the way the process is designed to work. For example, an organization is examining the length of time required by the emergency department to obtain a routine radiology report. The time may vary depending on how busy the radiology service is or by when the report is requested. On a particular day, there may be many concurrent requests for reports, making it difficult for the radiology department to fill one specific request. Or, the report may have been requested between midnight and 6:00 AM when fewer radiology technologists are on duty. Variation in the process of providing radiology reports is inherent, resulting from common causes such as staffing levels and emergency department census. A process that varies only because of common causes is said to be stable. The level of performance of a stable process or the range of the common-cause variation in the process can be changed only by redesigning the process. Common-cause variation is systemic and endogenous, that is, produced from within.

Another type of variation, *special-cause variation*, arises from unusual circumstances or events that may be difficult to anticipate and may result in marked variation and an unstable, intermittent, and unpredictable process. Special-cause variation is not inherently present in systems. It is exogenous, that is, produced from without, resulting from factors that are not part of the system as designed. Mechanical malfunction, intoxicated employees, floods, hurricanes, and other "acts of God" are examples of special causes

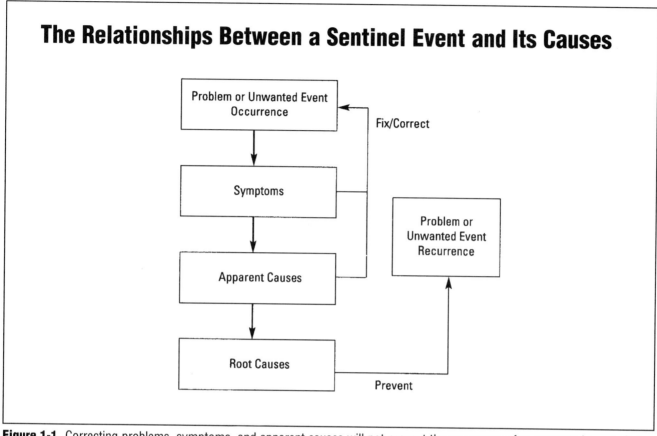

The Relationships Between a Sentinel Event and Its Causes

Figure 1-1. Correcting problems, symptoms, and apparent causes will not prevent the recurrence of an unwanted event. Only finding and resolving the root causes of the event can do this.
Source: Wilson PF, Dell LD, Anderson GF: *Root Cause Analysis: A Tool for Total Quality Management.* Milwaukee: ASQC Quality Press, 1993, p 11. Used with permission.

that result in variation. Special causes should be identified and mitigated or eliminated, if possible. However, removing a special cause will eliminate only that current abnormal performance in the process. It will not prevent the same special cause from recurring in the future. For example, firing an intoxicated employee who failed to monitor a secluded individual served or an overworked employee who was involved in a medication error will do little to prevent the recurrence of the same error. Instead, organizations should probe, understand, and address underlying common causes within their systems and processes such as personnel screening, staff education, staff supervision, information management, and communication.

Special causes in one process are usually the result of common causes in a larger system of which the process

is a part. For example, mechanical breakdown of a piece of equipment used during surgery may indicate a problem with an organization's preventive maintenance activities. Similarly, an intoxicated employee and understaffed units indicate a problem with the organization's screening and hiring practices. Human resources practices must be examined for common-cause problems involving personnel screening and interview processes.

In health care, all clinical processes are part of larger systems in the organization. Therefore, special-cause variation in performance that occurs in patient care is frequently the result of common causes in organization systems. This provides the opportunity to reduce the risk of a special cause in one process by redesigning the larger system of which it is a part.

Any variation in performance, including a sentinel event, may be the result of either a common cause, a special cause, or both. In the case of a sentinel event, the direct or proximate special cause could be uncontrollable factors. For example, a death results from a hospital's total loss of electrical power during a storm while an individual served is undergoing surgery. This adverse outcome is clearly the result of a special cause in the operating room that is uncontrollable by the operating room staff. Staff members may be able to do little to prevent a future power outage and more deaths. However, the power outage and resulting death can also be viewed as the result of a common cause in the organization's system for preparing for and responding to a utility failure and other emergencies. Perhaps the backup generator that failed was located in the basement, which flooded during the storm, and the organization had no contingency plan for this adverse situation.

When looking at the "chain of causation," proximate or direct causes tend to be nearest to the origin of the event. For example, the proximate causes of a medication error may include a deteriorated drug, product mislabeling or misidentification, or an improper administration technique. By contrast, root causes are systemic and appear far from the origin of the event, often at the foundation of the processes involved in the event. For example, root causes of a medication error might include communication problems, inadequate staff training, or poor competence assessment.

Most root causes alone are not sufficient to cause a failure; rather, the combination of root causes sets the stage. For example, both failure to communicate changes in the conditions of an individual served and failure to perform adequate assessments can be root causes of an individual's fall from his or her bed. Organizations that are successful in effectively identifying all of the root causes and their interactions can eliminate a plethora of risks when redesigning the processes.[5] Elimination of one root cause will reduce the likelihood of that one very specific adverse outcome occurring again. However, if the organization has missed the five other root causes, it is possible that they could interact to cause a different, but equally adverse, outcome. Chapter 5 describes how organizations can identify and explore the interrelationships of multiple root causes.

Benefits of Root Cause Analysis

Why conduct root cause analysis? All health care organizations experience problems of varying persistence and magnitude. Organizations can improve their operations and the care they provide through probing and addressing the roots of such problems. Individual accountability for "faulty" performance should not be the focus. Rather, the focus should be on systems—how to improve systems in order to prevent the occurrence of sentinel events or problems. This approach involves digging into the organization's systems to find new ways to do things. It is focused on answering the question, "What should we *do* to prevent this in the future?" not "What should we *have done* to prevent this from having occurred?" The emphasis is on improving systems of which clinical processes and people are but a part.

Thus, root cause analysis helps organizations identify risk or weak points in processes, underlying or systemic causes, and corrective actions. Moreover, information from root cause analyses shared between and among organizations can help to prevent future sentinel events. Knowledge shared in the health care field can contribute to proactive improvement efforts and results.

In addition, organizations use root cause analysis to meet Joint Commission requirements relating to the management of sentinel events. Each Joint Commission accreditation manual contains sentinel event requirements in the leadership and performance improvement chapters, which became effective January 1999. The requirements as they generally appear are shown in Sidebar 1-1, pages 10–11. Relevant leadership safety and error reduction requirements appear in Sidebar 1-2, page 12.

The sentinel event leadership requirement addresses what an organization should do when it experiences a sentinel event to ensure patient safety and comply with laws and regulations. The requirement gives the organization flexibility to define what would be considered a sentinel event within the organization. At a minimum, an organization's definition must include those events that are subject to review under the Sentinel Event Policy. The reporting requirements of any relevant agency should be considered by the organization in formulating its definition. Leaders must set the stage by establishing a culture conducive to performance improvement and must be involved in the process of identifying and managing sentinel events through root cause analysis. Leaders must also establish a plan to address improvement opportunities and identify who is responsible for implementing and assessing the plan.

The performance improvement requirements related to sentinel events necessitate well-designed processes, ongoing monitoring of performance (including data collection related to sentinel events), use of the finding(s) from analyses of sentinel events to design or redesign processes and identify changes that will improve performance or reduce the risk of sentinel events, and selection of performance measures for processes known to be associated with sentinel events in health care organizations. Root cause analysis, one vital technique in any performance improvement program, should be used with other programs and techniques.

Through these requirements, accredited organizations are expected to identify and respond appropriately to all sentinel events occurring in the organization or associated with services that the organization provides or provides for. An appropriate response includes conducting a thorough and credible root cause analysis, implementing improvements to reduce risk,

and monitoring the effectiveness of those improvements.

Finally, root cause analysis helps organizations meet information management requirements. The organization must determine whether its level of performance varies significantly and undesirably from what is expected or from that of other organizations. To do so, the organization should consider relevant literature, aggregated data, and comparative performance data and information, as specified in the information management chapter of accreditation manuals.

The Root Cause Analysis and Action Plan: Doing It Right

How can a health care organization ensure that its root cause analysis and action plan provide the "appropriate response" to a sentinel event occurring in the organization, as outlined in the requirements?

A root cause analysis is considered *acceptable* if it
- focuses primarily on systems and processes, not individual performance;
- progresses from special causes in clinical processes to common causes in organization processes;
- repeatedly digs deeper by asking "Why?"; then, when answered, asks "Why?" again, and so on;
- identifies changes that could be made in systems and processes—either through redesign or development of new systems or processes—that would reduce the risk of such events occurring in the future; and
- is thorough and credible.

Data gathered from review by the Joint Commission between January 1995 and March 2002 of more than 1,600 sentinel events indicate that nearly 80% of these events fall into 12 categories. These are suicide (in a 24-hour care facility); medication error; procedure complication; wrong-site surgery; delay in treatment; death in restraints; patient fall; elopement death; assault, rape, or homicide; transfusion death;

Sidebar 1-1. Joint Commission Sentinel Event Requirements

Leadership Requirements: The organization's leaders establish health care services that respond to community needs and needs of individuals served. The Joint Commission's accreditation requirements recognize that leadership is an important element in creating a framework for organizations to respond to sentinel events.

Leaders first and foremost are responsible for ensuring that the processes for identifying and managing sentinel events are defined and implemented. When a sentinel event occurs in a health care organization, appropriate individuals in the organization must be aware of the event, investigate and understand the causes that underlie the event, and make changes in the organization's systems and processes to reduce the probability of such an event in the future. Leaders are responsible for establishing processes for the identification, reporting, analysis, and prevention of sentinel events and for ensuring the consistent and effective implementation of a mechanism to accomplish these activities. They

- determine a definition of *sentinel event* and communicate this throughout the organization—the organization's definition must, at a minimum, include those events that are subject to review under the Joint Commission's Sentinel Event Policy and may include *near misses*;
- create a process for reporting of sentinel events within the organization and, as appropriate, to external agencies in accordance with law and regulation;
- create a process for conducting root cause analyses that are thorough, credible, and that focus on process and system factors; and

- determine a risk reduction strategy and action plan that includes measurement of the effectiveness of process and system improvements to reduce risk.

Improving Organization Performance Requirements: Organization performance improvement ensures that processes are designed well and systematically monitored, analyzed, and improved in order to enhance health care outcomes of individuals being served.

New or modified processes must be designed well at the outset. Good process design

- is consistent with the organization's mission, vision, values, goals and objectives, and plans;
- meets the needs of individuals served, staff, and others;
- is clinically sound and current (for instance, uses of practice guidelines, information from relevant literature, and clinical standards);
- is consistent with sound business practices;
- incorporates available information from other organizations about the occurrence of sentinel events to reduce the risk of similar sentinel events;
- includes analysis and/or pilot testing to determine whether the proposed change is an improvement; and
- incorporates the results of performance improvement activities.

Organizations should incorporate information related to these elements, when available and relevant, in the design or redesign of processes, functions, or services. Organizations collect data to monitor the

Sidebar 1-1. Joint Commission Sentinel Event Requirements (continued)

performance of processes that involve risks or may result in sentinel events. High-risk, high-volume, problem-prone areas related to the care, treatment, and service provided are monitored. Organizations select performance measures for processes that are known to jeopardize the safety of the individuals served or are associated with sentinel events in similar health care organizations.

Data are collected at the frequency and with the detail identified by the organization. Both the frequency and detail are appropriate for monitoring high-risk, problem-prone processes. Data are used to evaluate outcomes or performance of problem-prone processes. Organization staff intensively analyze undesirable patterns or trends in performance and sentinel events. The organization initiates intense analysis when the comparisons show that
- levels of performance, patterns, or trends vary significantly and undesirably from those expected;
- performance varies significantly and undesirably from that of other organizations;
- performance varies significantly and undesirably from recognized standards; or
- when a sentinel event has occurred.

Intense analysis involves studying a process to learn in greater detail about how it is performed or how it operates, how it can malfunction, and how errors occur. A root cause analysis is performed when a sentinel event occurs.

The occurrence of certain events should consistently elicit intense analysis. These include the following:

- Confirmed transfusion reactions;
- Significant adverse drug reactions;
- Significant medication errors and hazardous conditions; and
- Topics chosen by the leaders as performance improvement priorities and priorities for proactive reduction in patient risk, or when undesirable variation occurs that changes the priorities.

An intense analysis is also performed for the following:
- Major discrepancies, or patterns of discrepancies, between preoperative and postoperative (including pathologic) diagnoses, including those identified during the pathologic review of specimens removed during surgical or invasive procedures; and
- Significant adverse events associated with anesthesia use.

Organization staff identifies changes that will lead to improved performance and reduce the risk of sentinel events. The information from the data analysis is used to identify system changes that will improve performance or improve patient safety. Changes are identified based on the analysis of data from targeted study or from analysis of data from ongoing monitoring. A change is selected, and the organization plans to implement the change on a pilot test basis or across the organization. Performance measures are selected to determine the effectiveness of the change and whether it results in an improvement once it is implemented.

Sidebar 1-2. Leadership Requirements Relevant to Safety and Health Care Error Reduction

- The planning process provides for setting performance improvement priorities and identifies how the health care organization adjusts priorities in response to unusual or urgent events.

- Leaders and other relevant personnel collaborate in decision making.

- Leaders foster communication and coordination among individuals and departments.

- Leaders provide for mechanisms to measure, analyze, and manage variation in the performance of defined processes that affect patient safety.

- Leaders allocate adequate resources for measuring, assessing, and improving the organization's performance and for improving patient safety.

- Leaders assign personnel needed to participate in performance improvement activities and activities to improve patient safety.

- Leaders provide adequate time for personnel to participate in performance improvement activities and activities to improve patient safety.

- Leaders provide information systems and data management processes for ongoing performance improvement and improvement of patient safety.

- Leaders provide for staff training in the basic approaches to and methods of performance improvement and improvement of patient safety.

- Leaders assess the adequacy of their allocation of human, information, physical, and financial resources in support of their identified performance improvement and safety improvement priorities.

- Leaders measure and assess the effectiveness of their contributions to improving performance and improving patient safety.

- Leaders ensure implementation of an integrated patient safety program throughout the organization.

- Leaders ensure that an ongoing, proactive program for identifying risks to patient safety and reducing medical/health care errors is defined and implemented.

- Leaders ensure that patient safety issues are given a high priority and addressed when processes, functions, or services are designed or redesigned.

perinatal death or loss of function; and infant abduction or discharge to wrong family. Review of the root cause analyses of these events has allowed the Joint Commission to identify patterns for risk reduction activities.

Figure 1-2, page 14, shows the minimum scope of root cause analysis for ten specific types of sentinel events. An organization experiencing a sentinel event in one of these categories is expected to conduct a thorough and credible root cause analysis, which, at a minimum, inquires into each of the areas identified for that category of event. This inquiry should determine that there is, or is not, opportunity with the associated systems, processes, or functions to redesign or otherwise take action to reduce risk. A root cause analysis submitted in response to a sentinel event in one of the listed categories would be considered unacceptable if it did not address each of the areas specified for that type of event.

Detailed inquiry into these areas is expected when conducting a root cause analysis for the specified type of sentinel event. Inquiry into areas not checked (or listed) should be conducted as appropriate to the specific event under review.

To be *thorough*, the root cause analysis must include
- a determination of the human and other factors most directly associated with the sentinel event, and the process(es) and system(s) related to its occurrence;
- analysis of the underlying systems and processes through a series of "Why?" questions to determine where redesign might reduce risk;
- inquiry into each identified area for that category of event, for any event in one of the categories currently identified in the matrix of minimum requirements for root cause analysis (Figure 1-2), such that the organization can determine that there is, or is not, an opportunity within the associated processes to take actions to reduce risk;
- identification of risk points and their potential

contributions to this type of event; and
- a determination of potential improvement in processes or systems that would tend to decrease the likelihood of such events in the future, or a determination, after analysis, that no such improvement opportunities exist.

To be *credible*, the root cause analysis must
- include participation by the leadership of the organization and by the individuals most closely involved in the processes and systems under review;
- be internally consistent, that is, not contradict itself or leave obvious questions unanswered;
- provide an explanation for all findings of "not applicable" or "no problem;" and
- include consideration of any relevant literature.

All root cause analyses and action plans are considered and treated as confidential by the Joint Commission.

Due to the potential impact on the accreditation process, an organization should seek clarification of any questions about the Joint Commission's Sentinel Event Policy and the requirements for a root cause analysis by calling the Joint Commission's Sentinel Event Hotline (see Sidebar 1-3, page 15). Organizations may also wish to use the Joint Commission's Web site at www.jcaho.org, which includes detailed information on the Sentinel Event Policy and root cause analysis (see Sidebar 1-4, page 16).

Table 1-1, page 17, outlines the high-level key tasks involved in performing a thorough and credible root cause analysis and action plan. Overall, a thorough and credible root cause analysis should
- be clear (understandable information);
- be accurate (validated information and data);
- be precise (objective information and data);
- be relevant (focus on issues related or potentially related to the sentinel event);
- be complete (cover all causes and potential causes);
- be systematic (methodically conducted);
- possess depth (ask and answer all of the relevant

Minimum Scope of Root Cause Analysis for Specific Types of Sentinel Events

	Suicide (24° care)	Med. Error	Proced. Cmplic.	Wrong-site surg.	Treatmt. delay	Restraint death	Elopemnt. death	Assault/ rape/hom.	Transfusn. death	Infant abduction
Behavioral assessment process[1]	X					X	X	X		
Physical assessment process[2]	X		X	X	X	X	X			
Patient identification process		X		X					X	
Patient observation procedures	X					X	X	X	X	
Care planning process	X		X			X	X			
Continuum of care	X				X	X				
Staffing levels	X	X	X	X	X	X	X	X	X	X
Orientation and training of staff	X	X	X	X	X	X	X	X	X	X
Competency assessment/ credentialing	X	X	X		X	X	X	X	X	X
Supervision of staff[3]		X	X		X	X			X	
Communication with patient/family	X			X	X	X	X			X
Communication among staff members	X	X	X	X	X	X			X	X
Availability of information	X	X	X	X	X	X			X	
Adequacy of technological support		X	X							
Equipment maintenance/ management		X	X			X				
Physical environment[4]	X	X	X			X	X	X	X	X
Security systems and processes	X						X	X		X
Control of medications: storage/access		X							X	
Labeling of medications		X							X	

1 Includes the process for assessing patient's risk to self (and to others, in cases of assault, rape, or homicide where a patient is the assailant).

2 Includes search for contraband.

3 Includes supervision of physicians-in-training.

4 Includes furnishings, hardware (for example, bars, hooks, rods), lighting, and distractions.

Figure 1-2. The Joint Commission requires detailed inquiry into these areas when conducting a root cause analysis for the specified type of sentinel event. Inquiry into areas not checked (or not listed) should be conducted as appropriate for the specific event under review.

Sidebar 1-3. Sentinel Event Hotline

The Joint Commission established the Sentinel Event Hotline to respond to inquiries about the Sentinel Event Policy. For more information about the Hotline, visit www.jcaho.org/accredited+organizations/ hospitals/sentinel+events/index.htm. The Sentinel Event Hotline phone number is 630/792-3700. The hotline is staffed from 8:30 AM to 5:00 PM Central Standard Time, Monday through Friday.

Callers can

- speak with a member of the Joint Commission staff about the Sentinel Event Policy;
- request a sentinel event self-reporting form or a framework for a root cause analysis and action plan; and
- receive an update on the status of a sentinel event report submitted by the caller's organization.

"Why" questions); and

- possess breadth of scope (cover all possible systemic factors wherever they occur).

The product of a root cause analysis is an *action plan* that identifies the strategies the organization intends to implement to reduce the risk of similar events occurring in the future. The plan should address responsibility for implementation, oversight, pilot testing (as appropriate), time lines, and strategies for measuring the effectiveness of the actions.

An action plan will be considered *acceptable* if it

- identifies changes that can be implemented to reduce risk, or formulates a rationale for not undertaking such changes; and
- identifies who is responsible for implementation, when the action will be implemented (including any pilot testing), and how the effectiveness of the actions will be evaluated where improvement actions are planned.

The Joint Commission's framework for a root cause analysis and action plan appears as Figure 1-3, pages 18–20. This framework, to be used extensively in Chapters 4–6, provides a solid foundation for root cause analyses and action plans. The tool selection matrix, found in Chapter 7 as Figure 7-1 (page 142), can also be used as a guide to ensure that an organization considers and selects the most appropriate tools and techniques for root cause analysis.

References

1. Croteau RJ, Schyve PM: Chapter 7: Proactively error-proofing health care processes. In Spath P (ed): *Error Reduction in Health Care*. San Francisco: Jossey-Bass Publishers, 2000, pp 179–198.

2. Joint Commission Resources. *Failure Mode and Effects Analysis (FMEA): Proactive Risk Reduction*. Oakbrook Terrace, IL: 2002.

3. Brennan TA, et al: Incidence of adverse events and negligence in hospitalized patients. Results of the Harvard Medical Practice Study I. *N Engl J Med* 324(6):370–376, 1991.

4. Bates DW, et al: Incidence of adverse drug events and potential adverse drug events: Implications for prevention. *JAMA* 274(1):29–34, 1995.

5. Root cause analysis: Identifying multiple root causes is key to improving performance. *Jt Comm Perspectives on Patient Safety* 2: 4–5, Feb 2002.

Sidebar 1-4. Sentinel Event Information on the Web

The Joint Commission's Web site includes detailed information geared to helping health care organizations comply with the Joint Commission's Sentinel Event Policy. To access sentinel–event–related information from the Joint Commission's home page (www.jcaho.org), click on the "Accredited Organizations" icon and then click on the appropriate type of organization (such as Ambulatory Care, Behavioral Health Care, Hospitals, and so forth). Next, click on the "Sentinel Events" link that appears in the left-hand bar. This will take you to the "Sentinel Event Policy and Procedures." A bar on the left provides a list of other available information. Information, which can be downloaded, includes the following searchable topics:

- **Policy and Procedures:** A description of the Joint Commission's Sentinel Event Policy and procedures, including self-reporting and root cause analysis;

- **Sentinel Event Statistics:** Current statistical information on sentinel events by type, setting, source, outcome, and quarter, as well as by categories of root causes;

- **Voluntarily Reportable Sentinel Events:** Examples of sentinel events that are voluntarily reportable under the Joint Commission's Sentinel Event Policy;

- **Sentinel Event Advisory Group;**

- **Glossary:** Terms and definitions related to sentinel events;

- **Annotated Resources:** Joint Commission Resources products and general books and articles related to sentinel events;

- **Reporting Alternatives:** Alternatives for Sharing Sentinel Event Information with the Joint Commission: Four optional ways to provide the Joint Commission root cause analyses, actions plans, and other related information;

- *Sentinel Event Alert:* Newsletter about sentinel events, their causes, and error reduction strategies;

- **Position Statements:** Reporting of Medical/Health Care Errors: The Joint Commission's position statement;

- **Forms and Tools;** and

- **Organization Update Form.**

Table 1-1. Conducting a Root Cause Analysis and Implementing an Action Plan

- Assign a multidisciplinary team to assess the sentinel event.

- Establish a way to communicate progress to senior leadership.

- Create a high-level work plan with target dates, responsibilities, and measurement strategies.

- Define all the issues clearly.

- Brainstorm all possible or potential contributing causes and their interrelationships.

- Sort and analyze the cause list.

- For each cause, determine which process(es) and system(s) it is a part of and the interrelationships of causes.

- For each special cause, determine common cause(s).

- Begin designing and implementing changes while finishing the root cause analysis.

- Assess the progress periodically.

- Repeat activities as needed (for example, brainstorming).

- Be thorough and credible.

- Focus improvements on the larger systems.

- Redesign to eliminate the root cause(s) and the interrelationships of root causes that can create an adverse outcome.

- Measure and assess the new design.

A Framework for a Root Cause Analysis and Action Plan in Response to a Sentinel Event

Level of Analysis	Sentinel event	Questions	Findings	Root cause?	Ask "Why?"	Take action?
What happened?	Sentinel event	What are the details of the event? (Brief description)				
		When did the event occur? (Date, day of week, time)				
		What area/service was impacted?				
Why did it happen? — What were the most proximate factors? (Typically "special cause variations")	The process or activity in which the event occurred	What are the steps in the process, as designed? (A flow diagram may be helpful here)				
		What steps were involved in (contributed to) the event?				
	Human factors	What human factors were relevant to the outcome?				
	Equipment factors	How did the equipment performance affect the outcome?				
	Controllable environments factors	What factors directly affected the outcome?				
	Uncontrollable external factors	Are they truly beyond the organization's control?				
	Other	Are there any other factors that have directly influenced this outcome?				
		What other areas or services are impacted?				

This template is provided as an aid in organizing the steps in a root cause analysis. Not all possibilities and questions will apply in every case, and there may be others that will emerge in the course of the analysis. However, all possibilities and questions should be fully considered in your quest for "root causes" and risks reduction.

As an aid to avoiding "loose ends," the three columns on the right are provided to be checked off for later reference:

"Root Cause?" should be answered "yes" or "no" for each finding. A root cause is typically a finding related to a process or system that has a potential for redesign to reduce risk. If a particular finding that is relevant to the event is not a root cause, be sure that is addressed later in the analysis with a "Why?" question. Each finding that is identified as a root cause should be considered for an action and addressed in the action plan.

Ask "Why?" should be checked off whenever it is reasonable to ask why the particular finding occurred (or didn't occur when it should have)—in other words, to investigate further. Each item checked in this column should be addressed later in the analysis with a "Why?" question. It is expected that any significant findings that are not identified as root causes will have check marks in this column. Also, items that are identified as root causes will often be checked in this column, since many root causes themselves have "roots."

"Take Action?" should be checked for any finding that can reasonable be considered for a risk reduction strategy. Each item checked in this column should be addressed later in the action plan. It will be helpful to write the number of the associated Action Item in the "Take Action?" column for each of the Findings that require an action.

Figure 1-3. This framework outlines several questions that may be used to probe for systems problems underlying problematic processes. In each area, consider whether and how the factors can be improved, as well as the pros and cons of expending resources to make improvements.

Framework for a Root Cause Analysis (continued)

Level of Analysis	Questions	Findings	Root cause	Ask "Why?"	Take action?
Human resource issues	To what degree is staff properly qualified and currently competent for their responsibilities?				
	How did actual staffing compare with ideal levels?				
	What are the plans for dealing with contingencies that would tend to reduce effective staffing levels?				
	To what degree is staff performance in the operant process(es) addressed?				
	How can orientation and in-service training be improved?				
Information management issues	To what degree is all necessary information available when needed? accurate? complete? unambiguous?				
	To what degree is communication among participants adequate?				
Environmental management issues	To what degree was the physical environment appropriate for the processes being carried out?				
	What systems are in place to identify environmental risks?				
	What emergency and failure-mode responses have been planned and tested?				
Leadership issues: Corporate culture	To what degree is the culture conducive to risk identification and reduction?				
Encouragement of communication	What are the barriers to communication of potential risk factors?				
Clear communication of priorities	To what degree is the prevention of adverse outcomes communicated as a high priority? How?				
Uncontrollable factors	What can be done to protect against the effects of these uncontrollable factors?				

Why did that happen? What Systems and processes underlie those proximate factors? (Common-cause variation here my lead to special-cause variation in dependent processes)

→

Framework for an Action Plan in Response to a Sentinel Event

Risk Reduction Strategies	Person Responsible	Completion Date	Measures of Effectiveness
For each of the findings identified in the analysis as needing an action, indicate the planned action expected implementation date, and associated measure of effectiveness, OR…			
Action Item #1:			Measure:
If, after consideration for such a finding, a decision is made not to implement an associated risk reduction strategy, indicate the rationale for not taking action at this time.			
Action Item #2:			Measure:
Check to be sure that the selected measure will provide data that will permit assessment of the effectiveness of the action.			
Action Item #3:			Measure:
Consider whether pilot testing of a planned improvement should be conducted.			
Action Item #4:			Measure:
Improvements to reduce risk should ultimately be implemented in all areas where applicable, not just where the event occurred. Identify where the improvements will be implemented.			
Action Item #5:			Measure:
Action Item #6:			Measure:
Action Item #7:			Measure:
Action Item #8:			Measure:

Cite any books or journal articles that were considered in developing this analysis and action plan:

Chapter 2

Developing and Implementing a Policy and an Early Response Strategy for Sentinel Events

Root cause analysis plays a key role in the identification and prevention of sentinel events. What is a sentinel event and how does it differ from other events, incidents, or occurrences that take place routinely in health care organizations? What role does organization culture play in the identification and prevention of adverse events? What does the Joint Commission require when a sentinel event occurs? What types of events are reviewable by the Joint Commission and what types are nonreviewable? What types of events require root cause analysis? What issues should be considered as an organization develops its own sentinel event policy? What should an organization do following a sentinel event? Who must be notified? What are the legal and ethical considerations of disclosure to patients? The answer to some of these questions really is, "It depends." Although there are few hard-and-fast rules, some general guidelines can be useful. This chapter provides such guidelines while urging readers to consult additional sources of information as needed.

Sentinel Events and the Range of Adverse Events in Health Care

The Joint Commission defines *sentinel event* as an unexpected occurrence involving death or serious physical or psychological injury, or the risk thereof. Serious injury specifically includes loss of limb or function. The phrase *or the risk thereof* includes any process variation for which a recurrence would carry a

significant chance of a serious adverse outcome for a recipient of care, treatment, or service. Such events are called "sentinel" because they signal the need for immediate investigation and response. According to *Webster's*, the word *sentinel* means "one who watches or guards." An event is sentinel because it involves an unexpected variation in a process or an outcome and demands notice. Organizations must watch their care processes and guard against such an event.

Sentinel events commonly result from errors of commission or omission. An error of *commission* occurs as a result of an action taken, for example, when an improper technique is used to restrain an individual served and the individual served asphyxiates or when surgery is performed on the wrong limb. Other examples include a medication given by the incorrect route, an infant discharged to the wrong family, or electro-convulsive therapy administered to the wrong individual served.

An error of *omission* occurs when an action is *not* taken, for example, when a delayed diagnosis results in an individual's death, when a medication dose ordered is not given, when a physical therapy treatment is missed, or when a patient suicide is associated with a lapse in carrying out frequent observation. Errors of omission and commission may or may not lead to adverse outcomes. For example, a patient in seclusion is not monitored during the first two hours. The staff corrects the situation by beginning regular observations as specified in organization policy. The possibility of failure is present, however, and the mere fact that the staff does not follow organization policy regarding seclusion, and thereby violates acceptable professional standards, signals the occurrence of a failure requiring study to ensure that it does not happen again. In this case, the error of omission was insufficient monitoring. If the individual suffers serious physical or psychological harm during seclusion, the sentinel event is his or her adverse outcome. By definition, sentinel events require further investigation each time they occur.

Fortunately, the majority of failures, whether called events, incidents, or occurrences, cause no harm. For example, missed medication doses or doses administered at the wrong time rarely result in death or serious harm. Similarly, a missed observation of an individual served in seclusion rarely results in the individual's death or serious harm. However, the presence of these events may signal the presence of a much larger problem. Organizations should integrate information about such events as a part of their ongoing data collection and analysis.

Sometimes failures result in no serious harm but are significant enough to be considered a "near miss." For example, a drug dose is administered to an individual via the incorrect route, such as intravenously rather than orally. The individual feels the effect, but survives and suffers no permanent harm. However, the individual could have suffered harm, and perhaps would even be expected to with a similar error. It is good practice for organizations to conduct a root cause analysis or some other form of intensive analysis for such important single events, but such events usually are not reportable under the Joint Commission's Sentinel Event Policy described later in the chapter (see pages 23–24). Rather, the process used by the organization to review such events is evaluated during the organization's normal triennial survey.

Sentinel events—that is, important single events that should trigger intense investigation—are a subset of all adverse events. Of those sentinel events, an even smaller subset at the tip of the pyramid are the sentinel events that are reviewable under the Joint Commission's Sentinel Event Policy. These include failures involving patient deaths and permanent loss of function. Figure 2-1, page 23, shows the relationship of reviewable sentinel events to both sentinel events in general and broader categories of adverse events. Table 2-1, page 24, lists examples of sentinel events reviewable by the Joint Commission. See pages 26–27 for a complete description of reviewable sentinel events. As described in Chapter 1 (pages 10–11), organizations are required to conduct a thorough and credible root cause analysis and action plan for each of these sentinel events. The Joint Commission reviews the analysis and plan and adds the information to its database, to be described in more detail later. Table 2-2, page 24, provides a list of nonreviewable events.

Leadership, Culture, and Sentinel Events

Prior to developing and implementing a sentinel event policy, each organization needs to understand the role played by leaders and organization culture in the identification and prevention of adverse events.

Leaders must be deeply committed to performance improvement and to ensuring that members of their organization truly "live" their missions, visions, and values. They play a critical role in fostering an organization culture in which sentinel event reporting, root cause analyses, and proactive risk reduction are encouraged. Reporting helps the organization start the process of both identifying root causes and developing and implementing risk reduction strategies. Understanding that continuous improvement is essential to an organization's success, leaders must have the authority and willingness to allocate resources for root cause analyses and improvement initiatives. They must ensure that the processes for identifying and managing sentinel events are defined and implemented (see the leadership requirement in

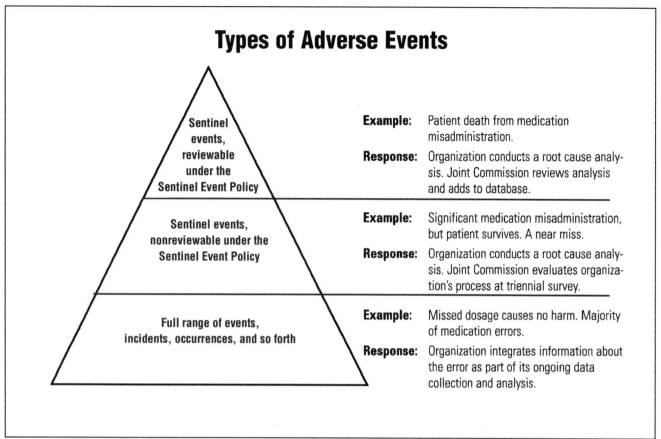

Types of Adverse Events

Sentinel events, reviewable under the Sentinel Event Policy	**Example:** Patient death from medication misadministration.
	Response: Organization conducts a root cause analysis. Joint Commission reviews analysis and adds to database.
Sentinel events, nonreviewable under the Sentinel Event Policy	**Example:** Significant medication misadministration, but patient survives. A near miss.
	Response: Organization conducts a root cause analysis. Joint Commission evaluates organization's process at triennial survey.
Full range of events, incidents, occurrences, and so forth	**Example:** Missed dosage causes no harm. Majority of medication errors.
	Response: Organization integrates information about the error as part of its ongoing data collection and analysis.

Figure 2-1. This triangular figure shows the relationship of Joint Commission–reviewable sentinel events to both sentinel events in general and the broader category of adverse events.

Sidebar 1-1, page 10). They must be willing and able to set an example for the organization and empower staff to identify and bring about necessary change. Effective leaders empower staff *throughout* the organization to acquire and apply the knowledge and skills needed to continuously improve processes and services.

Through commitment to performance improvement, patient safety, and proactive risk reduction, leaders build an organization culture that values change, creativity, teamwork, and communication. Teams provide much of the impetus for performance improvement. Communication and information flow throughout the organization in order to foster a barrier-free learning environment.

The Joint Commission's Sentinel Event Policy

When developing and implementing a sentinel event

policy of their own, organizations must understand the Joint Commission's Sentinel Event Policy. A description follows here. Figure 2-2, page 25, provides a graphic representation of the sentinel event process flow. The information provided here is current as of the date of publication. Changes to the policy are published in *Joint Commission Perspectives* and on the Perspectives homepage of the Joint Commission Resources Web site at www.jcrinc.com/perspectives. In support of its mission to improve the quality of health care provided to the public, the Joint Commission includes the reviews of organizations' activities in response to sentinel events in its accreditation process, including all full accreditation surveys and random unannounced surveys.

The four goals of the policy are to
• have a positive impact in improving care;

Table 2-1. Examples of Joint Commission–Reviewable Sentinel Events

- Any death, paralysis, coma, or other major permanent loss of function associated with a medication error.
- Any suicide of a patient in a setting where the patient is continuously housed, including suicides following elopement from such a setting.
- Any elopement, that is, unauthorized departure, of an individual from an around-the-clock care setting resulting in a temporally related death (suicide or homicide) or major permanent loss of function.
- Any procedure on the wrong patient, wrong side of the body, wrong organ, or wrong procedure.
- Any intrapartum (related to the birth process) maternal death.
- Any perinatal death, unrelated to a congenital condition, in an infant having a birth weight greater than 2,500 grams.
- Any assault, homicide, or other crime resulting in patient death or major permanent loss of function.
- A patient fall that results in death or major permanent loss of function as a direct result of the injuries sustained in the fall.
- A hemolytic transfusion reaction involving major blood group incompatibilities.
- A fire related to oxygen therapy provided by a durable medical equipment company in the home of an individual served that results in the individual's injury or death.
- An incident of cardiac arrest resulting in death or permanent injury to an individual undergoing an outpatient surgical procedure.

Table 2-2. Sentinel Events *Not* Reviewable by the Joint Commission

- Any "near miss."
- Full return of limb or bodily function to the same level as prior to the adverse event by discharge or within two weeks of the initial loss of said function.
- Any sentinel event that has not affected a recipient of care (patient, client, resident).
- Medication errors that do not result in death or major permanent loss of function.
- Suicide other than in an around-the-clock care setting or following elopement from such a setting.
- A death or loss of function following a discharge "against medical advice" (AMA).
- Unsuccessful suicide attempts *unless* resulting in major permanent loss of function.
- Unintentionally retained foreign body without major permanent loss of function.
- Minor degrees of hemolysis with no clinical sequelae.
- Note: In the context of its performance improvement activities, an organization may choose to conduct intensive assessment. For instance, an organization may perform root cause analyses for some nonreportable events.

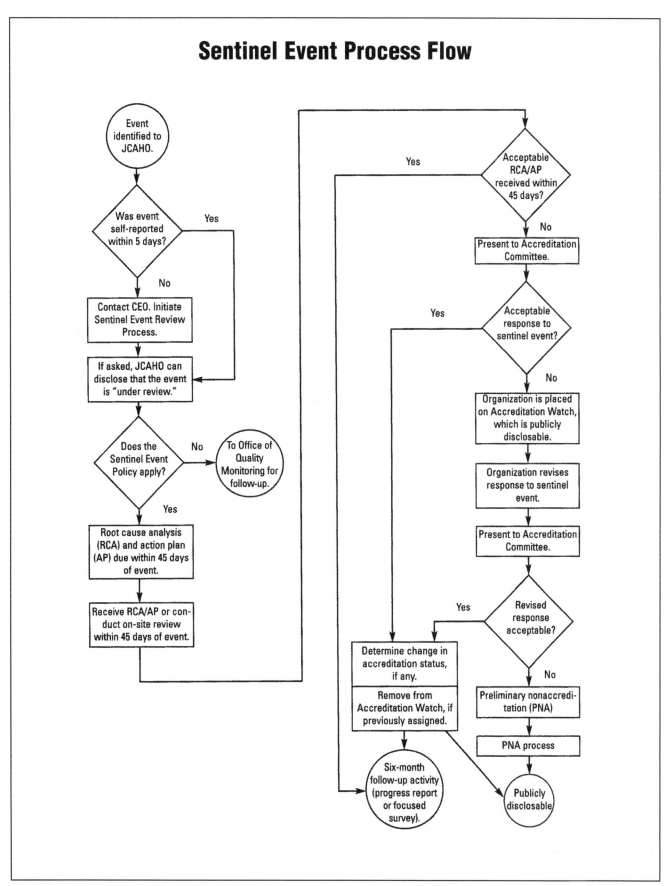

Figure 2-2. This flowchart displays the steps in the implementation of the Joint Commission's Sentinel Event Policy and its procedures.

- focus the attention of an organization that has experienced a sentinel event on understanding the causes that underlie that event, their interrelationships, and on making changes in the organization's systems and processes to reduce the probability of such an event in the future;
- increase the general knowledge about sentinel events, their causes, and strategies for prevention; and
- maintain the confidence of the public in the accreditation process.

Survey Process

In conducting an accreditation survey, Joint Commission surveyors will seek to evaluate the organization's compliance with the applicable requirements discussed in Chapter 1 and to score those requirements based on performance throughout the organization over time (for example, the preceding 12 months for a full accreditation survey). Under the sentinel event requirements, accredited organizations are expected to identify and respond appropriately to *all* sentinel events (as defined by the organization) occurring in the organization or associated with services that the organization provides, or provides for. Appropriate response includes conducting a timely, thorough, and credible root cause analysis, implementing improvements to reduce risk, and monitoring the effectiveness of those improvements.

Surveyors are instructed not to seek out specific sentinel events beyond those already known to the Joint Commission. The intent is to evaluate compliance with the relevant leadership and performance improvement requirements, that is, how the organization responds to sentinel events when they occur. However, if a surveyor becomes aware of a sentinel event while on–site, the organization will be required to provide follow-up information that indicates that a root cause analysis and action plan have been conducted. During a full accreditation survey, the surveyor will assess the organization's compliance with sentinel event–related requirements by

- reviewing documents that describe the organization's process for responding to a sentinel event;
- interviewing organization leaders and staff about their expectations and responsibilities for identifying, reporting, and responding to sentinel events; and
- asking for an example of a sentinel event that has occurred in the past year to assess the adequacy of the organization's process for responding to a sentinel event.

Surveyors will also review the effectiveness and sustainability of organization improvements in systems and processes in response to sentinel events previously evaluated under the Joint Commission's Sentinel Event Policy.

In selecting an example of a sentinel event, the organization may choose a "closed case" or a "near miss" to demonstrate its process for responding to a sentinel event. Additional examples may be reviewed if needed to more fully assess the organization's understanding of, and ability to conduct, a root cause analysis.

Reviewable Sentinel Events

The subset of sentinel events that falls within the scope of the Joint Commission's Sentinel Event Policy and is subject to review by the Joint Commission includes any occurrence that meets any of the following criteria:

- The event has resulted in an unanticipated death or major permanent loss of function,* not related to the natural course of the patient's illness or underlying condition;† or
- The event is one of the following (even if the

---

* *Major permanent loss of function* means sensory, motor, physiologic, or intellectual impairment not present on admission requiring continued treatment or lifestyle change. When major permanent loss of function cannot be immediately determined, applicability of the policy is not established until either the patient is discharged with continued major loss of function, or two weeks elapse with persistent major loss of function— whichever occurs first.

outcome was not death or major permanent loss of function unrelated to the natural course of the patient's illness or underlying condition):

○ Suicide of a patient in a setting where the patient receives around-the-clock care (for example, hospital, residential treatment center, crisis stabilization center);

○ Unanticipated death of a full-term infant;

○ Infant abduction or discharge to the wrong family;

○ Rape;††

○ Hemolytic transfusion reaction involving administration of blood or blood products having major blood group incompatibilities; and

○ Surgery on the wrong patient or wrong body part.§

The Joint Commission Web site (www.jcaho.org) has the most up-to-date information about options currently available for organizations that have experienced a sentinel event.

Again, Table 2-1, page 24, lists examples of reviewable sentinel events.

How the Joint Commission Becomes Aware of a Sentinel Event

Each health care organization is encouraged, but not required, to report to the Joint Commission any sentinel event meeting the above criteria for reviewable sentinel events. Alternatively, the Joint Commission may become aware of a sentinel event by some other means, such as communication from a patient, family member, employee of the organization, or through the media.

If the Joint Commission becomes aware (either through voluntary self-reporting or otherwise) of a sentinel event meeting the above criteria that has occurred in an accredited organization, the organization is expected to

• prepare a thorough and credible root cause analysis and action plan within 45 calendar days of the event or of becoming aware of the event; and

• submit to the Joint Commission its root cause analysis and action plan, or otherwise provide for Joint Commission evaluation of its response to the sentinel event under an approved protocol, within 45 calendar days of the known occurrence of the event.

The Joint Commission will then determine whether the root cause analysis and action plan are acceptable. If the root cause analysis or action plan is not acceptable, the organization is at risk for being placed on Accreditation Watch by the Accreditation Committee (see page 30). Joint Commission staff are available to consult with organizations about the thoroughness and credibility of the root cause analysis.

An organization that experiences a sentinel event that does *not* meet the criteria for review under the Sentinel Event Policy is still expected to complete a root cause analysis. However, the root cause analysis need *not* be made available to the Joint Commission.

---

† A distinction is made between an adverse outcome that is primarily related to the natural course of the patient's illness or underlying condition (not reviewed under the Sentinel Event Policy) and a death or major permanent loss of function that is associated with the treatment (including "recognized complications") or lack of treatment of that condition, or otherwise not clearly and primarily related to the natural course of the patient's illness or underlying condition (reviewable). In indeterminate cases, the event will be presumed reviewable and the organization's response will be reviewed under the Sentinel Event Policy according to the prescribed procedures and time frames without delay for additional information such as autopsy results.

†† *Rape*, as a reviewable sentinel event, is defined as unconsented sexual contact involving a patient and another patient, staff member, or unknown perpetrator while being treated or on the premises of the health care organization, including oral, vaginal, or anal penetration or fondling of the patient's sex organ(s) by another individual's hand, sex organ, or object. One or more of the following must be present to determine reviewability:
• Any staff-witnessed sexual contact as described above;
• Sufficient clinical evidence obtained by the organization to support allegations of unconsented sexual contact; and
• Admission by the involved individuals that sexual contact, as described above, occurred on the premises.

§ All events of surgery on the wrong patient or wrong body part are reviewable under the policy, regardless of the magnitude of the procedure.

Reasons for Reporting a Sentinel Event
to the Joint Commission

Although self-reporting of a sentinel event is not required, there are several advantages to the organization that reports a sentinel event, including the following:

- Reporting the event enables the addition of the "lessons learned" from the event and root cause analysis to be added to the Joint Commission's Sentinel Event Database, thereby contributing to the general knowledge about sentinel events and reducing risk for such events in many other organizations;
- Early reporting provides an opportunity for consultation with Joint Commission staff during the development of the root cause analysis and action plan; and
- The organization's message to the public that it is doing everything possible to ensure that such an event will not happen again is strengthened by its acknowledged collaboration with the Joint Commission to understand how the event happened and what can be done to reduce the risk of such an event in the future.

There is no difference in the expected response, time frames, or review procedures, whether the organization voluntarily reports the event or the Joint Commission becomes aware of the event by some other means.

Voluntary Reporting of Sentinel Events
to the Joint Commission

If an organization wishes to report an occurrence in the subset of sentinel events that are subject to review by the Joint Commission, the organization will be asked to complete a sentinel event reporting form (see Figure 2-3, page 29). This form can be accessed online at www.jcaho.org/accredited+organizations/ hospitals/sentinel+events/forms+and+tools/index.htm, by calling the Sentinel Event Hotline at 630/792-3700, or by calling the Office of Quality Monitoring at 630/792-5642.

The organization sends this form to the Joint Commission's Office of Quality Monitoring by mail or by facsimile (630/792-5636). The Office of Quality Monitoring can also be accessed online at www.jcaho.org/general+public/public+input/report+a+ complaint/off_qm.htm. Each organization is contacted within five days to finalize the due date, receive an incident number, and determine the method for which to review the root cause analysis and action plan.

Reviewable Sentinel Events That Are Not Reported
by the Organization

If the Joint Commission becomes aware of a sentinel event subject to review under the Sentinel Event Policy that was not reported to the Joint Commission by the organization, the chief executive officer of the organization is contacted, and a preliminary assessment of the sentinel event is made. For occurrences meeting the criteria for review under the Sentinel Event Policy, the organization is required to submit or make available an acceptable root cause analysis and action plan, or choose an approved protocol, within 45 calendar days of the event or becoming aware of the event.

Initial On-site Review of a Sentinel Event

An initial on-site review of a sentinel event is usually not conducted unless it is determined that there is a potential ongoing threat to patient health or safety or potentially significant noncompliance with major Joint Commission requirements. If an on-site ("for cause") review is conducted, the organization is billed an appropriate amount to cover the costs of conducting such a survey.

Disclosable Information

If, during the 45-day analysis period, the Joint Commission receives an inquiry about the accreditation status of an organization that has experienced a *reviewable* sentinel event, the

Joint Commission
on Accreditation of Healthcare Organizations

Accredited Organization Self-Reported Sentinel Event

_____

Full Name of Accredited OrganizationOrganization ID Number (HCO#)

_____

Street Address   City   State   Zip Code

_____

Date of Incident

Summary of Incident: (Please describe the event but do not include names of patient(s), caregiver(s), or other individual(s) involved in the event.)

_____

_____

_____

_____

_____

_____

_____

Select method of sharing sentinel event-related information:

_____ Mailing Root Cause Analysis

_____ Alternative #1   _____ Alternative #2

_____ Alternative #3   _____ Alternative #4

_____

Sentinel Event Contact (please print full name)   Phone #   E-mail address

_____

Title

_____

Signature   Date   Fax #

Figure 2-3. A Joint Commission–accredited organization that experiences a reportable sentinel event can complete this reporting form to apprise the Joint Commission of the event and the status of the root cause analysis.

organization's accreditation status is reported in the usual manner without making reference to the sentinel event. If the inquirer specifically references the sentinel event, the Joint Commission acknowledges that it is aware of the event and is working with the organization through the sentinel event review process.

Accreditation Watch Designation

Accreditation Watch is an attribute of an organization's Joint Commission accreditation status. It publicly acknowledges the collaborative efforts by the organization and the Joint Commission to understand the factors underlying a sentinel event and to implement appropriate changes to reduce the risk of such events in the future.

A health care organization is placed on Accreditation Watch when a reviewable sentinel event has occurred and has come to the Joint Commission's attention, and a thorough and credible root cause analysis of the sentinel event and action plan have not been completed within a specified time frame. Although Accreditation Watch status is not an official accreditation category, it can be publicly disclosed by the Joint Commission.

Required Response to a Reviewable Sentinel Event

If the Joint Commission becomes aware of a sentinel event in an accredited organization, and the occurrence meets the criteria for review under the Sentinel Event Policy, the organization is required to submit or otherwise make available an acceptable root cause analysis and action plan—or otherwise provide for Joint Commission evaluation of its response to the sentinel event using an approved protocol—within 45 calendar days of the event or of becoming aware of the event. If the determination that an event is reviewable under the Sentinel Event Policy is made more than 45 days following the known occurrence of the event, the organization will be allowed 15 days for its response.

If the organization fails to submit or otherwise make available an acceptable root cause analysis and action plan—or otherwise provide for Joint Commission

evaluation of its response to the sentinel event under an approved protocol—within the 45 calendar days (or within 15 calendar days, if the 45 days have already elapsed), the organization is at risk for being placed on Accreditation Watch if the sentinel event subsequently becomes known to the Joint Commission.

Initiation of Accreditation Watch

If the Joint Commission becomes aware that an organization has experienced a reviewable sentinel event, but the organization fails to submit or otherwise make available an acceptable root cause analysis and action plan—or otherwise provide for Joint Commission evaluation of its response to the sentinel event under an approved protocol—within 45 days of the event or of becoming aware of the event, a recommendation will be made to the Accreditation Committee to place the organization on Accreditation Watch. If the Joint Commission's Accreditation Committee places the organization on Accreditation Watch, the organization will then be permitted an additional 15 days to submit an acceptable root cause analysis and action plan or otherwise provide for Joint Commission evaluation of its response to the sentinel event under an approved protocol.

The organization will be offered assistance in performing a root cause analysis of the event. The Accreditation Watch status is considered publicly disclosable information. In all cases of an organization's refusal to permit review of information regarding a reviewable sentinel event in accordance with the Sentinel Event Policy and its approved protocols, the initial response by the Joint Commission is assignment of Accreditation Watch. Continued refusal may result in loss of accreditation.

Submission of Root Cause Analysis and Action Plan

The organization that experiences a sentinel event subject to review under the Sentinel Event Policy is asked to submit two documents: (a) the completed root cause analysis, which includes enough detail to demonstrate that the analysis is thorough and credible;

and (b) the resulting action plan that describes the organization's risk reduction strategies and plan for evaluating their effectiveness. A framework for a root cause analysis and action plan (see Figure 1-3, pages 18–20) is available to organizations as an aid in organizing the steps in a root cause analysis and developing an action plan. It is also available on the Joint Commission's Web site at www.jcaho.org.

The root cause analysis and action plan are *not* to include the patient's name or the names of caregivers involved in the sentinel event.

Reporting Options

If an organization self-reports the sentinel event to the Joint Commission, or if the Joint Commission becomes aware of a sentinel event at the organization, and the occurrence meets the criteria for review under the Sentinel Event Policy, the organization is required to submit or otherwise make available an acceptable root cause analysis and action plan—or otherwise provide for Joint Commission evaluation of its response to the sentinel event under an approved protocol—within 45 calendar days of the event or of becoming aware of the event.

Alternatively, if the organization has concerns about increased risk of legal exposure as a result of sending the root cause analysis documents to the Joint Commission, the following alternative approaches to Joint Commission review of the organization's response to the sentinel event are acceptable:

1. Review of root cause analysis and action plan documents brought to Joint Commission headquarters by organization staff, then taken back to the organization on the same day.
2. An on-site visit by a specially trained surveyor to review the root cause analysis and action plan. The organization will be assessed a charge sufficient to cover the average direct costs of the visit.
3. An on-site visit by a specially trained surveyor to review the root cause analysis and findings, without directly viewing the root cause analysis documents,

through a series of interviews and review of relevant documentation. For purposes of this review activity, "relevant documentation" includes, at a minimum, any documentation relevant to the organization's process for responding to sentinel events, and the action plan resulting from the analysis of the subject sentinel event. The latter serves as the basis for appropriate follow-up activity. The organization will be assessed a charge sufficient to cover the average direct costs of the visit.

4. Where the organization affirms that it meets specified criteria respecting the risk of waiving legal protection for root cause analysis information shared with the Joint Commission, an on-site visit by a specially trained surveyor to conduct interviews and review relevant documentation to obtain information about
   - the process the organization uses in responding to sentinel events, and
   - the relevant policies and procedures preceding and following the organization's review of the specific event, and the implementation thereof, sufficient to permit inferences about the adequacy of the organization's response to the sentinel event. In addition, the surveyor will conduct a standards-based evaluation of the patient care and organization management functions relevant to the sentinel event under review. The organization will be assessed a charge sufficient to cover the average direct costs of the visit.

A request for review of an organization's response to a sentinel event using any of these alternative approaches must be received by the Joint Commission within at least five days of the self-report of a reviewable event or of the initial communication by the Joint Commission to the organization that it has become aware of a reviewable sentinel event.

The Joint Commission's Response

Staff assesses the acceptability of the organization's response to the reviewable sentinel event, including the thoroughness and credibility of any root cause analysis information reviewed and the organization's action plan. If the root cause analysis and action plan are found to be thorough and credible, the response will be accepted and an appropriate follow-up activity will be assigned. A written report on progress related to the action plan is required by the six-month point.

If the response is unacceptable, staff will provide consultation to the organization on the criteria that have not yet been met and will allow an additional 15 calendar days beyond the original 45-day submission period for the organization to resubmit its response. This additional time is provided only if the organization's initial submission of its root cause analysis and action plan was within the 45-day time frame.

Depending on the nature and extent of the inadequacies of the organization's initial response to the sentinel event, the Joint Commission will determine whether an on-site visit should be made to assist the organization in conducting an appropriate root cause analysis and developing an action plan.

If, on review, the organization's response is still not acceptable, or the organization fails to respond, staff will recommend to the Accreditation Committee that the organization be placed on Preliminary Denial of Accreditation. If approved by the Accreditation Committee, this accreditation decision would be considered publicly disclosable information and the process for resolution of Preliminary Denial of Accreditation would be initiated.

When the organization's response, initial or revised, is found to be acceptable, the Joint Commission issues an *Official Accreditation Decision Report,* which reflects the Accreditation Committee's determination to (1) continue or modify the organization's current accreditation status and (2) terminate the Accreditation Watch if previously assigned; and assigns an appropriate follow-up activity, typically a written progress report or follow-up visit to be conducted within six months.

Follow-up Activity

The follow-up activity assesses, based on applicable standards, the organization's response to additional relevant information obtained since completion of the root cause analysis, the implementation of system and process improvements identified in the action plan, the means by which the organization continues to assess the effectiveness of those efforts, the organization's response to data collected to measure the effectiveness of the actions, and the resolution of any outstanding Type I recommendations (applicable to reporting option #4 described earlier). The follow-up activity is conducted when the organization believes it can demonstrate effective implementation—but no later than six months following receipt of the *Official Accreditation Decision Report.*

A decision to maintain or change the organization's accreditation status as a result of the follow-up activity or to assign additional follow-up requirements is based on existing decision rules unless otherwise determined by the Accreditation Committee.

Each sentinel event evaluated under the Joint Commission's Sentinel Event Policy is reviewed at the organization's next full accreditation survey. This review focuses on the implementation of risk reduction strategies and the effectiveness of these actions.

The Sentinel Event Database

To achieve the third goal of the Sentinel Event Policy—to increase the general knowledge about sentinel events, their causes, and strategies for prevention—the Joint Commission collects, aggregates, and analyzes data from the review of sentinel events, root cause analyses, action plans, and follow-up activities. These data and information form the content of the Joint Commission's Sentinel Event Database.

In response to concerns about potential increased legal exposure for accredited organizations through the sharing of such information with the Joint Commission, the Joint Commission has committed to the development and maintenance of this Sentinel Event Database in a fashion that excludes organization, caregiver, and patient identifiers. Three major categories of data elements are included in the Joint Commission's cumulative database:

- Sentinel event data (without organization, caregiver, or patient identifiers);
- Root cause data; and
- Risk reduction data.

Aggregate data relating to root causes and risk reduction strategies for sentinel events that occur with significant frequency will form the basis for future error-prevention advice to health care organizations through *Sentinel Event Alert* and other media.

Handling Sentinel Event–Related Documents

Upon completing the review of any submitted root cause analysis and action plan, and then abstracting the required data elements for the Joint Commission's Sentinel Event Database, the original root cause analysis documents are returned to the organization and all copies are shredded. Handling these sensitive documents is restricted to specially trained staff in accordance with procedures designed to protect the confidentiality of the documents.

The action plan resulting from the analysis of the sentinel event is initially retained to serve as the basis for the follow-up activity. Once the action plan has been implemented to the satisfaction of the Joint Commission, as determined through follow-up activities, the Joint Commission returns the action plan to the organization.

Legal Concerns over Confidentiality

The basic tenets of the Sentinel Event Policy are that an organization must perform a root cause analysis in response to a sentinel event and that it must share relevant root cause analysis information with the Joint Commission. Almost all organizations experiencing sentinel events appear to be moving quickly to address the first tenet. However, serious concerns regarding the potential discoverability of sentinel event–related information shared with the Joint Commission have created a significant barrier in meeting the second tenet for organizations in many states.

In response to these concerns, the Joint Commission has identified four alternative ways for a health care organization to report, and the Joint Commission to review, information regarding the organization's response to a sentinel event. These alternatives, outlined on page 31, are intended to reduce the exposure of sensitive sentinel event–related information while preserving an environment that encourages the candid and thorough assessment of the root causes of sentinel events. The Joint Commission believes that the confidentiality needs of accredited organizations can be well met by one or more of these alternatives. In the absence of new state or federal legislative protections, however, there are no absolute guarantees that these alternatives *ensure* the confidentiality of sentinel event–related information shared with the Joint Commission.

The Joint Commission firmly believes that the sharing of information between the Joint Commission and accredited organizations should not waive confidentiality protection granted to any particular information by any particular state law. If requested, the Joint Commission would strongly make this point in any court or legislature.

The Joint Commission has also identified two contractual arrangements that should substantively address the legal concerns regarding potential waiver of confidentiality protections in certain states. These arrangements involve having the health care organization either

- identify, through written agreement, the Joint Commission as a participating entity in the organization's peer review or quality improvement activities; or
- appoint the Joint Commission to the organization's peer review or quality improvement committee.

These arrangements clarify that the Joint Commission is *not* an external third party in the limited context of an intensive assessment of a sentinel event, and, therefore, no waiver of confidentiality protections has occurred by sharing sentinel event–related information with the Joint Commission. These arrangements, especially the former, may permit an organization to readily comply with the Sentinel Event Policy (that is, submit its root cause analysis and action plan to the Joint Commission) or otherwise serve to enhance the protections afforded by the four alternatives.

The wording of two sample agreement options is shown in Sidebar 2-1, right. The Joint Commission's General Counsel is available to answer questions or to negotiate state-specific modifications to the agreements. Find the General Counsel's contact information online at www.jcaho.org/contact+us/ directory.htm.

The Joint Commission is actively pursuing federal and state legislation to enhance protections for the confidentiality of sentinel event–related information shared with national accrediting bodies. Questions regarding legal protections of sentinel event information can be directed to the Department of Legal Affairs (contact information for the Department of Legal Affairs can be found online at www.jcaho.org/contact+us/directory.htm).

Developing a Sentinel Event Policy

The first step in developing an organization's sentinel event policy is to determine which events warrant root cause analysis. The Joint Commission expects accredited organizations to identify and respond appropriately to all sentinel events, as defined by the Joint Commission, occurring in the organization or associated with services that the organization provides, or provides for. This helps to ensure improvement of the organization's processes. As outlined earlier, appropriate response includes a thorough and credible root cause analysis, implementation of improvements to reduce risk, and monitoring of the effectiveness of those improvements.

Sidebar 2-1. Agreement Options for Safeguarding Confidentiality

Sample Ad Hoc Peer Review Committee Member Agreement

The (name of health care organization) and the Joint Commission agree that the accreditation process involves working together to improve the quality of health care, and that in carrying out that function the Joint Commission will serve as an ad hoc committee member of the (name of health care organization) peer review committee for those aspects of the accreditation process involving quality improvement initiatives. Such appointment to the peer review committee shall be limited to the review of information generated for said committee directly related to the Joint Commission requirements dealing with quality improvement and to the guidance furnished by the Joint Commission with respect to quality improvement initiatives.

Sample Consultant Relationship Agreement

The (name of health care organization) and the Joint Commission agree that the accreditation process involves working together to improve the quality of health care, and that in carrying out that function the Joint Commission will serve as a consultant to the (name of health care organization) peer review committee for those aspects of the accreditation process involving quality improvement initiatives. Such consulting service to the peer review committee shall be limited to the review of information generated for said committee directly related to the Joint Commission requirements dealing with quality improvement and to the guidance furnished by the Joint Commission with respect to quality improvement initiatives.

The new leadership requirement (outlined in Chapter 1, page 10) requires each accredited organization to define *sentinel event* for its own purposes in establishing mechanisms to identify, report, and manage these events. While this definition must be consistent with the Joint Commission's general definition of *sentinel event* as provided on page 21, accredited organizations have some latitude in setting more specific parameters to define *unexpected, serious,* and *the risk thereof*.

For example, an organization may wish to define a sentinel event as a serious event involving staff and visitors as well as patients. Or an organization may wish to include
- all unusual events, even though they may result in only minor adverse outcomes;
- all events that must be reported to an external agency; or
- events with potential for an adverse public, economic, or regulatory impact.

At a minimum, an organization's definition must include those events that are subject to review under the Sentinel Event Policy (see pages 26–27). The definition must also apply organizationwide and must appear in writing in an organization plan or policy. Through a collaborative process, organization leaders, including medical, nursing, and administrative staff, should develop the definitions or categories of events that warrant root cause analysis.

In developing the organization's sentinel event policy, leaders may also address the process for reporting a sentinel event to leadership, how near misses are to be handled, and the ongoing management of sentinel events and prevention efforts. Leaders may also want to identify
- the individual responsible for receiving initial notification of a sentinel event;
- the individual responsible for assessing whether or not the event warrants an in-depth root cause analysis based on the organization's definition of a

sentinel event (this may be the same individual, for example, a physician, risk manager, quality assurance coordinator, or program manager);
- how this individual communicates the need for in-depth investigation and necessary information to a team of individuals responsible for performing the root cause analysis; and
- the individual responsible for facilitating and overseeing a team-based root cause analysis process.

Leaders should also address confidentiality, discoverability, and disclosure. Information obtained during the investigation of sentinel events through root cause analysis or other techniques is often highly sensitive. The organization's sentinel event policy must address how confidentiality will be protected. The policy should also address the procedure for obtaining legal consultation to protect relevant documents such as meeting minutes, reports, and conversations from discovery in the event of a future lawsuit. The policy must be clear on whether the state in which the organization operates protects the details of a sentinel event investigation from discovery under the organization's quality management, peer review, or risk management programs.

Following development of the organization's sentinel event policy, leaders should ensure that all staff and physicians are educated about the policy and procedures. In-service programs and new staff and physician orientation must address the organization's sentinel event policy on a regular and continuing basis. Table 2-3, page 36, outlines the steps described in this section.

Early Response Strategies

An organization has just experienced a sentinel event leading to a serious adverse outcome. What must be done?

Following the occurrence of a sentinel event, staff members must simultaneously take a number of actions. An organization's sentinel event policy should outline early response strategies. These include

---

Table 2-3. Steps in Developing a Sentinel Event Policy

- Define *sentinel event,* setting specific parameters for what constitutes *unexpected, serious,* and *the risk thereof* (remember that the general definition must be consistent with the Joint Commission's definition).

- Include the definition of *sentinel event* in writing in an organization plan or policy.

- Determine which events warrant root cause analysis using a collaborative process.

- Determine the process for reporting a sentinel event to leadership.

- Determine the process for reporting the event to external agencies.

- Determine how near misses are to be handled.

- Determine how the ongoing management of sentinel events and prevention efforts are to be handled.

- Address how confidentiality of information related to sentinel events will be protected.

- Address the procedure for obtaining legal consultation to protect relevant documents.

- Educate all staff and physicians about the policy and procedures; ensure ongoing education.

- Review the policy annually and revise information, such as reviewable sentinel events, process for reporting sentinel events, confidentiality issues, legal issues, and relevant staff education, as appropriate.

- providing prompt and appropriate care for the affected patient(s);
- containing the risk of an immediate recurrence of the event; and
- preserving the evidence.

Appropriate Care

The prompt and proper care of an individual served who has been affected by a sentinel event should be the providers' and staff members' first concern following the event. Care could involve, as appropriate, stabilizing the individual, arranging for his or her transportation to a health care facility for surgery or testing, providing medications, taking actions to prevent further harm, and reversing the harm that has occurred, if possible. When appropriate, physicians should obtain medical consultation related to the

adverse event and arrange to receive necessary follow-up information.

Communication with the family (discussed further on pages 38 and 40–41) is vital during the time period immediately following the event.

Risk Containment

Immediately following a sentinel event, the organization must respond by immediately containing the risk of the event from occurring again. If an individual suffered a stroke as a result of the misadministration of a drug, are other individuals at risk for similar injuries? If so, the organization must take immediate action to safeguard such individuals served from a repetition of the unwanted occurrence. Risk management texts, articles appearing in the literature, and associations such as the American Society for Healthcare Risk Management* can provide detailed guidance.

Preservation of Evidence

To learn from a failure and understand why it occurred, it is critical to know exactly what occurred. Preserving the evidence is essential to this process. Immediate steps should be taken to secure any biological specimens, medications, equipment, medical or other records, and any other material that might be relevant to investigating the failure.[1] In medication-related events, syringes of recently used medications and bottles of medications should be preserved and sequestered. Because such evidence may be discarded as a part of routine operations, such as when empty vials are thrown into trash cans, it is critical to obtain and preserve it promptly. Protocols established by the health care organization should specify the steps to be taken to preserve relevant evidence following a sentinel event.

Event Investigation

Documentation and appropriate communication and disclosure to relevant parties must also be considered immediately following the occurrence of a sentinel event.

Documentation

Proper medical record documentation of errors or sentinel events is critical for the continuity of care. Documentation tips appear in Table 2-4, page 38. A thoroughly completed incident reporting form can be very helpful during the early stages of event investigation and during steps 2 through 4 of root cause analysis (Chapters 3 and 4). Health care organizations use a variety of occurrence or incident reporting tools and generally have a policy and procedure covering their use. Forms or questionnaires may be general in nature, covering all types of adverse events, or be specific to event types. Figure 2-4, page 39, is a sample medication error occurrence report.

Communication and Disclosure

With the occurrence of a sentinel event, personnel involved in the incident should promptly notify those responsible for error reporting and investigation within the organization. Supervisors, quality and risk management professionals, and administrators should be informed. These individuals can determine how best to notify other parties, including the press and external agencies such as federal, state, and local authorities. Legal counsel should be sought early in the process. Counsel can provide guidance in how to discuss the situation with the family, how to prevent disclosure of potentially libelous information, and how to handle media relations.[2]

One recommendation states that organizations maintain two lists of key people to contact following a sentinel event: key individuals *within* the organization and individuals *outside* the organization.[3] Both lists should be kept up to date with current telephone numbers and should be accessible to managers, supervisors, and members of a crisis management team. A sample sentinel event notification checklist appears as Figure 2-5, page 40.

Responding to media queries through organization protocols will help to avert complications related to patient confidentiality, legal discovery, and heat-of-the-moment coverage.[4] Notification requirements should be reflected in organization policies and procedures. These should include policies for communication with the individual served and family, described below.

A provider's communication and disclosure with relevant parties following the occurrence of an event that led or could have led to patient injury is critical. Relevant parties include

- individuals served and families affected by the event;

---

* The American Society for Healthcare Risk Management can be found online at www.ashrm.org or by phone ar 312/422.3980.

Table 2-4. Tips for Documenting Adverse Events

- Assign the most involved and knowledgeable member(s) of the health care team to record factual statements of the event in the patient's record.

- Record any medical follow-up completed, planned, or needed.

- Avoid writing information in the medical record that is unrelated to the care of the patient (such as "legal office notified").

- Avoid writing derisive comments about other providers—in the event of a disagreement with another clinician, the health care team should document only the basis for their treatment recommendations.

- When adding information to the patient's record after an adverse event has occurred, mark the entry with the actual date it is written; do not "backdate" any entries.

- Beware of creating entries that appear self-serving—especially explanations intended solely to justify someone's actions.

Source: Keyes C: Responding to adverse events. *Forum* 18(1):3, 1997. Used with permission

- colleagues who could provide clarification, support, and the opportunity to learn from the error;
- the health care organization's and individual provider's liability insurers;
- appropriate organization staff, including risk managers or quality assurance representatives; and
- others who could provide emotional support or problem-solving help.

Conferring with other members of the care team following an adverse event enables the provider to clarify factual details and the proper sequence of what occurred. It can also help to identify what needs to be done in response to the event.

A Joint Commission safety and health care error reduction requirement indicates that the responsible licensed independent practitioner (LIP) or his or her designee clearly explains the outcome of any treatments or procedures to the patient and, when appropriate, the family, whenever those outcomes differ significantly from the anticipated outcomes. This means that

individuals served and, when appropriate, their families, must be informed about the outcomes of care, including unanticipated outcomes, such as a sentinel event.

Good communication between providers and patients is instrumental in achieving positive care outcomes. Yet health care professionals often do not tell patients or families about their mistakes. Fear of malpractice litigation and the myth of perfect performance reinforce poor provider communication of errors to patients and their families. There is little doubt that the current malpractice crisis is a deterrent to the openness required for quality improvement.[5] However, errors not communicated to patients, families, fellow staff members, and organizations are errors that do not contribute to systems improvement.

Disclosing mistakes to patients and their families is difficult, at best. Yet legal and ethical experts generally advise practitioners to disclose mistakes to individuals served and their families in as open, honest, and forthright a manner as possible. One suggestion is that

Sample Medication Error Occurrence Report

Today's Date:_____ Reported By:_____

Completed By:_____

Initials of staff member filling medication:_____

Initials of staff member checking medication:_____

Date of incident:_____

Patient name:_____ Date of birth:_____

Location:_____

Circle all items that describe medication error occurrence:
1. Wrong medication
2. Incorrect dose of medication
3. Incorrect dosage form
4. Wrong patient
5. Incorrect label
6. Delivered to wrong patient
7. Clinical judgment error (for example, failure to properly evaluate drug interaction screen, approval of medication for use in a patient whose disease state contraindicates the use of the drug)

Explain:_____

_____

Briefly describe the incident, outlining all known factual information:

_____

_____

_____

Results of occurrence (circle all that apply):
1. Error discovered before medication taken
2. Medication taken:_____ Number of doses:_____
3. No apparent patient injury
4. Patient injury:

Explain:_____

_____

Change in process or education to avoid error from occurring in the future:

Figure 2-4. Unlike a general form or questionnaire, this sample medication error occurrence report exemplifies a form specific to medication errors.

Source: Lynn Moran, RPh, BS, Grove City, OH. Used with permission.

Sentinel Event Notification Checklist

SENTINEL EVENT

OCCURRENCE: _____

DATE AND TIME: _____

CONTACT PERSON: _____

Chief Executive Officer

Name: _____

Office Phone Number: _____

After-hours Phone Number: _____

Name/Phone of Designated Backup: _____

Notified by: _____

Date and Time: _____

Results of Contact: _____

Chief Nursing Officer

Name: _____

Office Phone Number: _____

After-hours Phone Number: _____

Notified by: _____

Date and Time: _____

Results of Contact: _____

Medical Staff Director

Name: _____

Office Phone Number: _____

After-hours Phone Number: _____

Notified by: _____

Date and Time: _____

Results of Contact: _____

Risk Manager

Name: _____

Office Phone Number: _____

After-hours Phone Number: _____

Notified by: _____

Date and Time: _____

Results of Contact: _____

Legal Counsel

Name: _____

Office Phone Number: _____

After-hours Phone Number: _____

Notified by: _____

Date and Time: _____

Results of Contact: _____

Public Relations Director

Name: _____

Office Phone Number: _____

After-hours Phone Number: _____

Notified by: _____

Date and Time: _____

Results of Contact: _____

Chair, Board of Directors

Name: _____

Office Phone Number: _____

After-hours Phone Number: _____

Notified by: _____

Date and Time: _____

Results of Contact: _____

Figure 2-5. This checklist can be used as a guide to properly notify the relevant officers following the occurrence of a sentinel event. Fill in the appropriate names and phone numbers and keep the information in a location readily accessible to managers and supervisors. The list should be periodically reviewed and updated.

Source: Adapted from Spath P: Avoid panic by planning for sentinel events. *Hosp Peer Rev* 23(6):117, 1998. Used with permission.

physicians have an ethical obligation to tell individuals served about significant medical errors when such disclosure would

- benefit the health of the individual served;
- show respect for the individual's autonomy; or
- be called for by principles of justice.[6]

This idea maintains that disclosure of a mistake may foster learning by compelling the physician to acknowledge it truthfully and that the physician-patient relationship can be enhanced by honesty.[7] Disclosing a mistake might even reduce the risk of litigation, in fact, if the patient appreciates the physician's honesty and fallibility as a fellow human being. Another study reports that the risk of litigation nearly doubles when patients are not informed by their physicians of moderately serious mistakes.[8] Physician guidelines in disclosing medical mistakes to patients are offered by yet another report.[9] Sidebar 2-2, pages 42–43, outlines practical issues a physician may encounter in disclosing an error to a patient or his or her family. Please note that these are guidelines about issues to consider, not Joint Commission requirements. Organizations should be aware that the disclosure of an error or event requires individualized handling. Risk management or legal counsel should be involved in communication with the patient and his or her family.

Onward with Root Cause Analysis

Having developed and implemented a sentinel event policy, the organization is now ready to start performing root cause analyses and developing an action plan. The next four chapters present in a step-by-step, workbook format how to perform a root cause analysis and develop, implement, and assess an improvement-driven action plan.

References

1. Perper JA: Life-threatening and fatal therapeutic misadventures. In Bogner MS (ed): *Human Error in Medicine*. Hillsdale, NJ: Lawrence Erlbaum Associates, 1994, p 33.

2. Spath P: Avoid panic by planning for sentinel events. *Hosp Peer Rev* 23(4):117, 1998.

3. Spath, p 117.

4. Keyes C: Responding to adverse events. *Forum* 18(1):2–3, 1997.

5. Blumenthal D: Making medical errors into … "medical treasures." *JAMA* 272(23):1867–1868, 1994.

6. Wu AW, et al: To tell the truth: Ethical and practical issues in disclosing medical mistakes to patients. *Gen Intern Med* 12(12):770–775, 1997.

7. Wu AW, McPhee SJ: Education and training: Needs and approaches for handling mistakes in medical training. Presented at the Examining Errors in Health Care Conference, Rancho Mirage, CA, Oct 13–15, 1996.

8. Witman AB, Hardin S: Patients' responses to physicians' mistakes. *Forum* 18(4):4–5, 1997.

9. McPhee SJ, et al: Practical issues in disclosing medical mistakes to patients. Presented at the Examining Errors in Health Care Conference, Rancho Mirage, CA, Oct 13–15, 1996.

Sidebar 2-2. Practical Issues for Physicians in Disclosing Medical Mistakes to Patients

Medical Mistakes Requiring Disclosure

A medical mistake is a commission or an omission with potentially negative consequences for the patient that would have been judged incorrect by skilled and knowledgeable peers at the time it occurred.

Deciding Whether to Disclose a Mistake

In general, a physician has an obligation to disclose clear mistakes that cause significant harm that is remediable, mitigable, or compensable. In cases in which disclosing a mistake seems controversial, the decision should not be left to the individual physician's judgment.* It is important to obtain a second opinion to represent what a reasonable physician would do and be willing to defend in public. This second opinion is best obtained from an institution's ethics committee or quality review board rather than from informal consultation with peers.

Timing of Disclosure

Disclosure should be made as soon as possible after the mistake occurred but at a time when the patient is physically and emotionally stable.

Who Should Disclose the Mistake?

When a mistake is made by a physician in training, responsibility is shared with the attending physician. It may be most appropriate for the attending and house

officer to disclose the mistake to the patient together. When a mistake is made by a practicing physician, he or she should disclose the mistake to the patient. When the mistake results from the system of medical care delivery, it may be appropriate to involve an institutional representative in the disclosure, such as an administrator, risk manager, or quality assurance representative.

What to Say?

Disclosure is often difficult, for technical as well as emotional reasons. The facts of the case may be too complicated to be explained easily and may not be known precisely. The physician may be tempted to frame the disclosure in a way that obscures that a mistake was made. In telling the patient about an error, the physician should do the following:

- Treat it as an instance of "breaking bad news" to the patient;
- Begin by stating simply that he or she regrets that he or she has made a mistake or error;
- Describe the decisions that were made, including those in which the patient participated;
- Describe the course of events, using nontechnical language;
- State the nature of the mistake, consequences, and corrective action taken or to be undertaken;

---

* A Joint Commission safety and error reduction requirement states that the responsible licensed independent practitioner or his or her designee inform the individual served (and when appropriate, the family of the individual served) about the outcomes of care, including unanticipated outcomes.

Sidebar 2-2. Practical Issues for Physicians in Disclosing Medical Mistakes to Patients (continued)

- Express personal regret and apologize for the mistake;
- Elicit questions or concerns from the patient and address them; and
- Ask if there is anyone else in the family to whom he or she should speak.

Consequences of Disclosure

Physicians are most often concerned about the potentially harmful consequences of disclosing a mistake—particularly the risk of a lawsuit. Serious mistakes may come to light even if the physician does not disclose them. Any perception that the physician tried to cover up a mistake might make patients angry and more litigious. The risks inherent in disclosing a mistake may be minimized if

- patients appreciate the physician's honesty;
- patients appreciate that physicians are fallible;
- disclosure is prompt and open;
- disclosure is made in a manner that diffuses patient anger;
- sincere apologies are made;
- charges for associated care are forgone; and
- a prompt and fair settlement is made out of court.

Disclosure of Mistakes Made by Other Physicians

A physician may encounter situations where he or she recognizes that a colleague physician has made a mistake. That colleague may choose to disclose the mistake or not. The physician recognizing the mistake has the following options:

- Wait for the other physician to disclose the mistake;
- Advise the other physician to disclose the mistake;
- Simultaneously advise quality assurance or risk management;
- Arrange a joint meeting to discuss the mistake; and
- Tell the patient directly of the error.

The physician may be reluctant to disclose a colleague's error due to

- lack of definitive information;
- fear of hurting the colleague's feelings;
- fear of straining a professional relationship;
- fear of a libel suit;
- the sense that he or she could easily have made the same error ("There but for the grace of God go I"); and
- social norms against "tattling" on peers.

Source: Adapted from McPhee SJ, et al: Practical issues in disclosing medical mistakes to patients. Paper presented at the Examining Errors in Health Care Conference, Rancho Mirage, CA, Oct 13–15, 1996.

Chapter 3
Preparing for Root Cause Analysis

Step 1: Organize a Team
Step 2: Define the Problem
Step 3: Study the Problem
Step 4: Determine What Happened
Step 5: Identify Contributing Process Factors
Step 6: Identify Other Contributing Factors
Step 7: Measure—Collect and Assess Data on Proximate and Underlying Causes
Step 8: Design and Implement Interim Changes
Step 9: Identify Which Systems Are Involved—The Root Causes
Step 10: Prune the List of Root Causes
Step 11: Confirm Root Causes and Consider Their Interrelationships
Step 12: Explore and Identify Risk Reduction Strategies
Step 13: Formulate Improvement Actions
Step 14: Evaluate Proposed Improvement Actions
Step 15: Design Improvements
Step 16: Ensure Acceptability of the Action Plan
Step 17: Implement the Improvement Plan
Step 18: Develop Measures of Effectiveness and Ensure Their Success
Step 19: Evaluate Implementation of Improvement Efforts
Step 20: Take Additional Action
Step 21: Communicate the Results

This first workbook chapter describes how to prepare for a root cause analysis. It covers organizing a team, defining the problem, and studying the problem. The information is presented in a practical and user-friendly way. To help illustrate the steps of root cause analysis, sentinel events involving a suicide, elopement, treatment delay, and medication error are described as examples throughout this and subsequent chapters. A description of each incident of a sentinel event appears in Sidebar 3-1, pages 46–47. Checklists and worksheets are presented throughout the chapter. Use this and the following three chapters as a workbook—fill in the blanks.

A sentinel event or a near miss has occurred in an organization. Leadership has been informed and, in the case of an actual sentinel event, an organization has completed preliminary response procedures, including ensuring patient safety, risk containment, and prevention of repeat action (see Chapter 2, pages 35–37). The appropriate staff members have documented the event and ensured communication with appropriate stakeholders.

1 Step One: Organize a Team

The first step involved in conducting a root cause analysis might be to assign a team to assess the sentinel event or potential sentinel event. Leaders must lay the groundwork by creating an environment conducive to root cause analysis and improvement through team initiatives. Often, leaders will need to assure staff that organization improvement through the identification and reduction of risks, rather than the assignment of blame, is the objective.

Sidebar 3-1. Sentinel Event Examples

Suicide

The Incident: A 20-year-old male is admitted for observation to the behavioral health care unit of a general hospital. He has a well-documented history of depression. On his second day in the unit, he attends a particularly clamorous group session. Following the session, he commits suicide in his bathroom by hanging himself from the showerhead with bedding sheets.

The Time: between 10:00 AM and 11:00 AM. A registered nurse finds him at 11:05 AM, calls a code, and starts unsuccessful resuscitation efforts.

Elopement

Nursing staff in a long term care facility note that an 80-year-old woman with a history of progressive dementia is unusually irritable and restless. She is pacing, talking in a loud voice, and complaining about a number of issues. The nurses on duty are unable to appease her or to determine the cause of what they view as a "bad mood." Staff members frequently remind the woman to move away from the exit door. In the evening, the staff discover that the woman is no longer on the unit, nor in the building. The woman left the facility without warm clothing on a cold evening with subzero temperatures. She is found dead the following morning in a wooded area near the facility. Death was caused by exposure.

Treatment Delay

A 60-year-old woman goes to an ambulatory health care organization to receive her annual physical from her long-time physician. The physician gives the woman a prescription for an annual mammogram, which she schedules for two weeks later. Following the mammogram, the woman is informed that she will hear from her physician's office. A week later, a nurse in the physician's office calls the woman and informs her that additional mammogram views are required. The nurse does not express the physician's wish that the tests be done immediately nor that there is a potential health problem. Required to perform extra duties because of short staffing, the nurse files the X-ray reports in the woman's medical record rather than in the proper file for tests requiring follow-up.

The woman does not forget the need for a follow-up mammogram and calls the physician's office to ascertain whether a repeat mammogram has been ordered. Another office employee assumes that if the woman did not get a call from the physician directly, the woman has nothing to worry about and should relax. The woman does not question the employee's answer, nor tell her about the nurse's call, and attempts to think no more about it.

Several weeks later, the woman calls the physician's office again, noting that she can feel a hard lump in her breast and mentioning that it hurts. The physician tells her to come into the office right away. Upon review of her record, the physician finds the results and orders another mammogram with needle localization "Stat." The woman has the test, which identifies a change in the size of a nodule from a previous mammogram. This

Sidebar 3-1. Sentinel Event Examples (continued)

requires an immediate biopsy, which is positive. Subsequent surgery reveals that the cancer has metastasized.

Medication Error

A 60-year-old man receiving home care services complains about a headache to his home health nurse on each of the nurse's three visits during a one-week period. The man indicates that he is tired of "bothering" his primary care physician about various symptoms. At the conclusion of the third visit, the nurse offers to discuss the man's complaint with his primary care physician upon return to the agency. When the nurse discusses the headache with the man's physician, the physician instructs the nurse to call the local pharmacy with the following prescription:

    Fioricet Tabs. #30
    Sig: 1-2 tabs q 4-6 hours prn headache
    Refill x3

In error, the nurse telephones the pharmacy

and provides the following prescription:

    Fiorinal Tabs. #30
    Sig: 1-2 tabs q 4-6 hours prn headache
    Refill x3

The man has a long history of peptic ulcer disease, which resulted in several hospitalizations for gastrointestinal bleeding. The man began taking the Fiorinal, which contains 325 mg aspirin per tablet. In contrast, the intended medication—Fioricet— contains 325 mg acetaminophen per tablet.

The man completes the entire first prescription and 15 tablets of the first refill. At this point, he goes to the emergency department with acute abdominal pain, blood in the stool, and a hemoglobin of 4.9. He is immediately admitted to the intensive care unit. Within hours, he needs life support. After several units of blood and a four-week hospital stay, the man recovers and is able to return to his home following this "near miss" sentinel event.

Guilt, remorse, fear, and anxiety are common emotions felt by staff following the occurrence of a sentinel event. These emotions must be addressed and discussed at the earliest stages of team formation. Leaders must put staff members at ease so that staff can contribute to risk reduction. Leaders further lay the groundwork by empowering the team to make changes or recommendations for changes, providing the resources (including time to do the work), and ensuring a defined structure and process for moving forward. See Checklist 3-1, page 48.

What Is a Team?

Webster's defines the word *team* as a number of individuals associated with one another. *Team* implies a group that is dynamic and working together toward a well-defined goal. In the health care environment, a team should be multidisciplinary. Unlike committees that meet for a long period of time for an ongoing purpose, a team generally meets on an ad hoc basis for shorter periods of time. Once a specific project is completed, the team often disbands—with a sense of accomplishment.

Checklist 3-1. Essential Elements for a Team Go-ahead

While developing a team and selecting team members, ensure that the following three elements are present in the organization's leadership:

☐ Awareness of and support from top leadership;

☐ Leadership commitment to provide necessary resources, including time; and

☐ An empowered team with authority and responsibility to recommend and implement process changes.

Checklist 3-2. Team Composition

While drawing up a tentative list of team members, check to ensure that the team includes

☐ individuals closest to the event or issues involved;

☐ individuals critical to implementation of potential changes;

☐ a leader with a broad knowledge base, who is respected and credible;

☐ someone with decision-making authority; and

☐ individuals with diverse knowledge bases.

Why Use a Team?

A team approach brings increased creativity, knowledge, and experience to solving a problem. Multidisciplinary teams distribute leadership and decision making to all levels of the organization. Teams in health care organizations provide a powerful way to integrate services across the continuum of care.[1] They also provide a powerful and often successful way to effect systemwide improvement.

Who Should Work on the Team?

A team may be established on an ad hoc basis, or, if the relevant disciplines or services are represented, the core of an appropriate team may already exist in the form of a targeted performance improvement team or some other type of team. The selection of team members is critical. The team should include staff at all levels closest to the issues involved—those with fundamental knowledge of the particular process involved. These individuals are likely to be those with the most to gain from improvement initiatives. The team should also include an individual with some distance from the process, but who possesses excellent analytical skills. The team should also include at least one individual with decision-making authority as well

as individuals critical to the implementation of anticipated changes. Team members should bring to the table a diverse mix of knowledge bases and should be knowledgeable about and committed to performance improvement. See Checklist 3-2 above.

Organizations may also wish to think "outside the box" in terms of possible team members. Might a former individual served, family member, or other community member be able to provide a unique perspective and valuable input? For example, perhaps the town's retired pharmacist or a former patient that experienced a near miss sentinel event could be invited to join the root cause analysis team. If one of the suspected root causes of a sentinel event relates to information management, perhaps a member of the local chapter of an information management association or organization could be invited.

Team composition may need to change as the team moves in and out of areas within the organization that affect or are affected by the issues being analyzed. An organization should allow for and expect this to happen. However, the core team members should remain as stable as possible throughout the process, at least in terms of leadership and areas or functions represented. Realistically, the selection of all team members cannot take place until the broad aim of the improvement initiatives to be generated by the root cause analysis and improvement action plan are identified.[2]

For example, a team investigating the cause of the death of an individual served due to a fall from bed might include representatives from nursing, medicine, education, physical and recreational therapy (to help look at new ways of designing processes), plant safety, leadership, and infection control (to assist in devising an acceptable environmental solution). A description of possible members of teams examining the sentinel events described in Sidebar 3-1 follows.

The core team investigating the **suicide** in a behavioral health care unit might include the following individuals: nurse(s) from the behavioral health unit; an occupational therapist, physical therapist, or recreation therapist (who has clinical skills and knowledge, but would not necessarily spend much time on the behavioral health care unit); a social worker on the unit; a representative from the education department; a psychiatrist (who attended the patient); a medical staff leader who understands processes and has the authority to change medical staff policy; the manager of the behavioral health unit; a representative from quality improvement or risk management (who will act as the facilitator); an administrative representative at the vice president level (such as nursing, patient care, or an associate VP) who can make changes; a safety engineer; and a safety consultant (on an ad hoc basis).

The core team investigating the **elopement** of a resident from a long term care facility might include the following individuals: the director of nursing; a unit nurse (regular care provider); a nursing assistant (who regularly cared for the resident); the medical director; the safety director or person responsible for the safety program; the individual responsible for performance

improvement (facilitator of group); a social service worker; and a unit activity staff member.

The core team investigating the **treatment delay** in an ambulatory care organization might include the following individuals: the director of the ambulatory care organization; a staff physician; the medical director; the appointments scheduler; a staff nurse; the staff educator; the office manager; the manager of the laboratory used by the organization; the pharmacy supplier used by the organization; and the director or manager of quality/performance improvement.

The core team investigating a **medication error** in a home health agency might include the following individuals: a home health nurse; a nursing supervisor; an agency director or administrator; a member of pharmacy supplier's staff; a local pharmacist (ad hoc); the medical director; the quality/performance improvement coordinator; and an information technology or management staff member, as available.

To have a significant effect in a health care organization, performance improvement must address clinical care. The participation of physicians and other medical staff members on root cause analysis and improvement teams is critical. Leaders must understand the barriers to medical staff involvement and take steps to overcome those barriers.[3]

The team should have a leader who is knowledgeable, interested, and skilled at group consensus building and applying the tools of root cause analysis. This person

---

Tip: Team Size

Core teams limited in size to fewer than ten individuals tend to perform with greater efficiency. Experts needed at different points can be added as ad hoc team members and attend only the relevant meetings.

guides the team through the root cause analysis process while encouraging open communication and broad participation. The leader may function as a facilitator, or a separate team member can be assigned to play the facilitator role. This individual should be skilled at being objective and moving the team along. It is best if the leader and facilitator are not "stakeholders" in the processes and systems being evaluated.

Ad hoc members who can provide administrative support, additional insight, and resources should be identified as well. Use Worksheet 3-1, page 64, to indicate proposed team members.

At the first team meeting, the leader should establish ground rules that will help the team avoid distractions and detours on the route to improvement. The following ground rules provide a framework that will allow the team to function smoothly:

- *Team mission*: The leader should establish the group's mission or focus as one of systems improvement rather than individual fault finding.
- *Decision making:* The group must decide what kind of consensus or majority is needed for a decision, recognizing that decisions belong to the entire team.
- *Attendance*: Attendance is crucial. Constant late arrivals and absences can sabotage the team's efforts. Set guidelines for attendance.
- *Meeting schedule:* For high attendance and steady progress, the team should agree on a regular time, day, and place for meetings. These matters should be revisited at various times during the team's life.
- *Opportunity to speak:* By agreeing at the outset to give all members an opportunity to contribute and to be heard with respect, the team will focus its attention on the important area of open communication.
- *Disagreements*: Similarly, the team must agree to disagree. It must acknowledge and accept that members will openly debate differences in viewpoint. Discussions may overflow outside the

meeting room, but members should feel free to say in a meeting what they say in the hallway.
- *Assignments*: The team should agree to complete assignments within the particular time limits so that delayed work from an individual does not delay the group.
- *Other rules*: The team should discuss all other rules that members feel are important. These can include whether senior management staff can drop in, whether pocket pagers should be checked at the door, what the break frequency is, and so forth.

See Sidebar 3-2, page 51, for techniques team leaders or facilitators can use to ensure high-quality group discussion.

Step Two: Define the Problem

One of the first steps taken by the root cause analysis team is to define the problem—that is, to describe, as accurately as possible, what happened or what nearly happened. The purpose of defining the problem as clearly and specifically as possible is to help focus the team's analysis and improvement efforts. If the team defines and understands the problem clearly, much time, effort, and a great deal of frustration can be saved.

Tool: *Brainstorming*

In response to a sentinel event, the team might ask, "What actually happened or what created the 'red flag' warning of the occurrence of a sentinel event?" Initially, the problem or event can be defined simply, such as the following:

- Surgery performed on the incorrect site;
- Patient committed suicide by hanging;
- Individual served died following overdose of drug; or
- Fire killed individual in restraints.

These simple statements focus on what happened or the outcome, not on why it happened. During later steps in the root cause analysis process, the team will focus on the sequence of events, on the "whys," and on contributing factors.

For near misses or improvement opportunities, the problem statements above could be restated as follows:
- Surgery was almost performed on the incorrect site;
- Patient attempted to commit suicide by hanging;
- Individual served received overdose of drug but survived without long-term consequences; or
- Fire could have killed restrained individuals.

Use Worksheet 3-2, page 65, to define the problem.

Particularly in the event of a near miss, multiple problems may be present. Which problem should be selected first for analysis? Each team needs to develop ranking criteria to help meet this challenge. One

option is to rank problems by their cost impact, organization priority, consequence or severity, safety impact, or real or potential hazard.[4] Each problem should be addressed one at a time. The highest-ranked problem should be tackled and solved before initiating work on lower-ranked problems. This topic will be explored in more depth in Chapter 6.

Tool: *Multivoting*

Help with Problem Definition

The information disseminated from the Joint Commission's Sentinel Event Database can be helpful in an organization's identification of a problem or area for analysis. The purpose of this database is to increase general knowledge about sentinel events, their causes, and strategies for prevention. The Joint Commission collects and analyzes data from the review of actual sentinel events, root cause analyses, action plans, and follow-up activities in all types of health care organizations. By sharing the "lessons learned" with other health care organizations, the hope is that the risk of future sentinel events will be reduced. Organizations can learn about sentinel events that occur with significant frequency, their root causes, and possible risk reduction strategies through the Joint Commission's publication *Sentinel Event Alert* (see Sidebar 3-3, page 52) and the newsletter *Joint Commission Perspectives* received by the CEO of every accredited organization. All organizations can use the areas or problems outlined here as a starting point in the identification of a problem area for analysis. Table 3-1, page 53, lists the most frequently reviewed sentinel events by the Joint Commission. Sentinel events

Tip: Criteria for a Well-Defined Problem
A well-defined problem statement states what is wrong and focuses on the outcome, not why the outcome occurred.

Sidebar 3-3. *Sentinel Event Alert*

The following topics have been covered in the Joint Commission's *Sentinel Event Alert* publication:

- Prevention of treatment delays (Jun 2002);
- Prevention of ventilator-related deaths and injuries (Feb 2002);
- Prevention of wrong-site surgery (Dec 2001, Aug 1998);
- Prevention of medication errors (Sep 2001, May 2001, Feb 2001, Nov 1999, Feb 1998);
- Prevention of needlestick and sharps injuries (Aug 2001);
- Prevention of medical gas mix-ups (Jul 2001);
- Prevention of exposure to Cruetzfeldt-Jakob disease (Jun 2001);
- Prevention of fires in the home care setting (Mar 2001);
- Prevention of adverse events related to infusion pumps (Nov 2000);
- Prevention of falls (Jul 2000);
- Prevention of operative and postoperative complications (Feb 2000);
- Prevention of blood transfusion errors (Aug 1999);
- Prevention of infant abductions (Apr 1999);
- Prevention of restraint deaths (Nov 1998); and
- Prevention of inpatient suicides (Nov 1998).

Current and past issues of *Sentinel Event Alert* can be found on the Joint Commission's Web site at www.jcaho.org/about+us/ news+letters/sentinel+event+alert/index.htm.

---

process or system that are susceptible to failure or system breakdown. They generally result from a flaw in the initial design of the process or system, a high degree of dependence on communication, nonstandardized processes or systems, and failure or absence of backup.

For example, risk points during the medication use process include interpretation of an illegible order by a pharmacist and the time during which a registered nurse mixes the medication dose to administer to an individual served. In surgical procedures requiring the use of lasers, a risk point occurs during the use of anesthetic gases which, if not properly synchronized with use of the laser, can ignite and cause fires. During preoperative procedures, verification of the body side and part constitutes a risk point.

Tool: *Brainstorming*

Identification of failure-prone systems yields problem areas requiring focus through root cause analysis. A number of factors increase the risk of system failures, including complexity—the high number of steps and handoffs in work processes. Complex systems may be dynamic, with constant change and tight time pressure and constraints. The "tight coupling" of process steps can increase the risk of failure. Tightly coupled systems or processes do not provide much slack or the opportunity for recovery. Sequences do not vary and delays in one step throw off the entire process. Variable input and process steps that are nonstandardized can also increase the risk of process failure. So can processes carried out in a hierarchical rather than team structure.

reported in the national media can also serve as a source of ideas for problem analysis.

Identification of risk points can often yield a helpful problem list. *Risk points* are those specific places in a

For example, medication ordering is frequently cited as a risk-prone system due to organization hierarchies. Nurses and pharmacists may be reluctant to question physicians writing the orders. Some organization cultures, in fact, may create a hierarchical rather than team structure for the entire medication use process. Similarly, verification of surgical sites by surgical team members can suffer from hierarchical pressures. Nurses may be reluctant to question physicians. Language barriers coupled with a hierarchical culture can present a particularly dangerous scenario. Worksheet 3-3, page 66, can be used to identify risk-prone systems in an organization.

Most frequently, sentinel events result from multiple system failures. They also frequently occur at the point where one system overlaps or "hands off" to another. An organization should be tracking high-risk, high-volume, and problem-prone processes as part of its performance improvement efforts. High-risk, high-volume, problem-prone areas will vary by organization and will be integrally related to the care, treatment, and service provided. For example, to reduce the risk of infant abductions, a large maternity unit will want to focus on its infant-parent identification process. To reduce the risk of patient suicide, a behavioral health care unit will want to focus on its suicide risk assessment process. The list of frequently occurring sentinel events published by the Joint Commission (see Table 3-1, right), the organization's risk management data, morbidity and mortality data, performance data (including sentinel event indicators and aggregate data indicators), or information about problematic processes generated by field-specific or professional organizations can provide starting places to find such processes.

At a minimum and as required by the Joint Commission's performance improvement requirements, a team should look at the following processes as appropriate to the care and services provided:

- Medication use;
- Operative and other procedures that place individuals at risk;
- Use of blood and blood components;
- Restraint use;
- Seclusion when it is part of the care or services provided;

Table 3-1. Types of Sentinel Events Reviewed by the Joint Commission

Since establishing its Sentinel Event Database in 1995, the Joint Commission has tracked the frequency of occurrence of various types of sentinel events. The following events appear most frequently in the database:

- Patient suicide;
- Medication error;
- Operative or postoperative complications;
- Wrong-site surgery;
- Delay in treatment;
- Patient death or injury in restraints;
- Patient elopement;
- Assault, rape, or homicide;
- Patient fall;
- Infant abduction/discharge to wrong family;
- Transfusion error;
- Fire;
- Medical equipment–related event;
- Anesthesia-related event;
- Death associated with patient transfer;
- Maternal death;
- Perinatal death/loss of function; and
- Ventilator death/injury.

- Care or services provided to high-risk populations; and
- Staffing effectiveness.

Tool: *Brainstorming*

Developing a Preliminary Work Plan and Reporting Mechanism

After a team has chosen a problem for analysis and defined the problem, it can develop a preliminary work plan for investigating the sentinel event through root cause analysis. The plan should outline the overall strategy, key steps, individuals responsible for each step, target dates, and reporting mechanisms.

To develop the overall strategy, a team can articulate what it is trying to accomplish. This is the aim statement. An aim statement can be sharpened[5] by completing the sentences found in Worksheet 3-4, page 67. A specific aim statement answers the question: "What are we trying to accomplish?" It should be objective and measurable. Possible aim statements for the investigation of each example sentinel event described in Sidebar 3-1, pages 46–47, follow.

The aim statement for the **suicide** investigation might read as follows:

> Our aim is to improve the quality of suicide risk assessment on admission. The process begins when the individual served is admitted to the behavioral health care unit (or, it might begin in an emergency department, therapist's office, and so forth, before the individual is admitted) and ends with an appropriate assessment of suicide risk and the individual's placement at the appropriate level of care. By working on this process, we expect to enhance the effectiveness of suicide risk assessment and achieve appropriate risk assessments with 98% to 100% of our admissions. We must work on this process to reduce the risk of patient suicide.

The aim statement for the **elopement** investigation might read as follows:

> Our aim is to improve the quality of assessment of residents for possible risk for elopement. The process begins with the initial assessment of at-risk status when the resident is admitted to the facility, continues through regular reassessment during the resident's stay, and ends only when the resident is discharged from the facility or passes away. By working on this process, we expect to enhance the effectiveness of initial risk assessment and achieve ongoing risk reassessment with 99% to 100% of our residents. We must work on this process to reduce the risk of resident elopement.

The aim statement for the **treatment delay** investigation might read as follows:

> Our aim is to improve processes that reduce the risk of sentinel events associated with treatment delays. The processes must begin with leadership definition of appropriate staffing levels and the provision of high-quality initial orientation for staff members. The processes include regular assessment of ongoing staff competence and ongoing assessment of staffing needs. By working on these processes, we expect to enhance the effectiveness of initial orientation and ongoing competence assessment with 90% to 100% of staff members achieving assessment scores of 90% or higher on all posttraining tests. We must work on this process to reduce the risk of treatment delays associated with insufficient staff orientation and training or insufficient staffing.

The aim statement for the **medication error** investigation might read as follows:

> Our aim is to improve the effective communication of information related to medication orders. The process begins when the home health care nurse receives the physician's instructions to order a medication and ends with the accurate administration of the right drug to the right individual, in the right dosage, at the right time, with the right frequency, using the right administration technique, and via the right route. By

improving the process for communicating critical medication-related information, we expect to enhance the accuracy and timeliness of medications administered by our nurses to home care patients and therefore decrease adverse medication occurrences by 10% in each of the next five years. We must work on this process to reduce the likelihood of injury or death due to medication errors.

The creation of a detailed work plan is critical to the process and to securing management support. A plan outlining target dates for accomplishing specific objectives provides a tool against which to guide and measure the team's progress.

The full work plan should include target dates for major milestones and key activities in the root cause analysis process. These can mirror the steps of the root cause analysis and action plan itself, including

- defining the event and identifying the proximate and underlying causes;
- collecting and assessing data about proximate and underlying causes;
- designing and implementing interim changes;
- identifying the root causes;
- planning improvement; and
- testing, implementing, and measuring the success of improvements.

Checklist 3-3, page 56, indicates the key steps to include in a work plan for a root cause analysis. Each activity is described further in later chapters. Use Worksheet 3-5, page 68, to outline key steps, individuals responsible, and target dates for a root cause analysis. Also outline the reporting mechanisms and use the checklist portions to double-check overall strategy and report quality.

Tool: *Gantt chart*

A team's outline of the reporting mechanism aims to ensure that the right people receive the right information at the right time. At the beginning of the process, the team leader or facilitator should establish a means of communicating team progress and findings to senior leadership. Keeping senior leaders informed on a regular basis is critical to management support of the root cause analysis initiative and implementation of its recommendations. Although it is difficult to provide guidelines on how *a regular basis* should be defined, because this varies widely depending on circumstances, communication with senior leaders should increase in frequency with

- serious adverse outcomes;
- repeated adverse events;
- events requiring solutions from multiple parts of the organization;
- possible solutions requiring the investment of significant amounts of money; and
- the media's involvement in the case and its solutions.

Frequency of communication also will vary according to the actions required in the short term to prevent recurrence of the event. Communication frequency should be weighed against the speed with which information emerges from the investigation. If information is emerging rapidly, the team leader should give thought to the most productive timing for communication. A description of reporting considerations for each of the sample root cause analysis investigations follows.

The reporting mechanism for the **patient suicide** investigation should ensure that the psychiatrist on the team is providing his or her colleagues with regular updates on the team's progress at clinical department meetings. This will prepare the medical staff for recommended policy changes. Similarly, at executive staff meetings, the vice president on the team should be providing the CEO, chief operating officer, and other leaders with regular updates on the team's progress. Communication should be frequent in order to foster

Checklist 3-3. Key Steps in Root Cause Analysis and Improvement Planning

The work plan can include the following key activities with target dates for each major milestone.

☐ Organize a team   Completion date: _____

☐ Define the problem   Completion date: _____

    ☐ Choose area(s) for analysis

    ☐ Develop a plan

☐ Study the problem   Completion date: _____

    ☐ Gather information

☐ Determine what happened and why (proximate causes)   Completion date: _____

    ☐ Identify process problem(s)

    ☐ Determine which patient care processes are involved

    ☐ Determine factors closest to the event

    ☐ Extract measurement data

☐ Identify root causes   Completion date: _____

    ☐ Determine which systems are involved

☐ Design and implement an action plan for improvement

    ☐ Identify risk reduction strategies   Completion date: _____

        ☐ Formulate actions for improvement
        (considering actions, measures, responsible
        party, desired completion date, and so forth)

        ☐ Consider the impact of the improvement action

    ☐ Design improvements   Completion date: _____

    ☐ Implement action plan   Completion date: _____

    ☐ Measure effectiveness   Completion date: _____

        ☐ Develop measures of effectiveness

        ☐ Assure success of measurement

    ☐ Evaluate implementation efforts   Completion date: _____

    ☐ Communicate results   Completion date: _____

Note: *In preparing a root cause analysis in response to a sentinel event that is reviewable by the Joint Commission, remember that the analysis must be completed no more than 45 days after the event's occurrence or becoming aware of the event.*

leadership acceptance of future recommendations, particularly those involving significant resources.

The reporting mechanism for the **resident elopement** investigation should ensure that the safety director is providing the facility management and operations staff with regular updates on the team's progress. This will prepare them for any recommended building alterations to enhance the safety of the care environment.

The reporting mechanism for the **treatment delay** investigation in an ambulatory care organization should ensure that the office manager is keeping the physician/medical director informed of the team's progress on a regular basis. This will prepare the medical director for any changes that might be warranted with respect to staffing levels and staff orientation, training, and ongoing competence assessment.

The reporting mechanism for the **medication error** investigation should ensure that the information technology (IT) staff member is keeping his or her colleagues informed of the team's progress. This will facilitate the smooth integration of any new processes or technology that may be recommended to enhance safe medication ordering.

3 Step Three: Study the Problem

The team is now ready to start studying the problem. This involves collecting information surrounding the event or near event. Time is of the essence, because key facts can be forgotten in a matter of days. In fact, the individual closest to the event or near event may have already collected some information that the team can use as a starting point. Often a written statement provided by individuals involved in the event and prepared as near the time of the event as possible can be useful throughout the root cause analysis process. At times, the individual(s) closest to the event may withhold critical information due to the fear of blame. The team should consider

how to eliminate such fear. It may be necessary in some instances to obtain the individual's written statement and then proceed without his or her contribution in the early stages of the analysis.

Early on, the team should give thought to how information is to be recorded. Some methods are more suitable than others. For example, audiotaping or videotaping an interview with someone intimately involved with the event is likely to increase the individual's defensiveness. Note taking is an effective way to record interviews. Videotapes, drawings, and/or photographs are also effective media to record physical evidence. For instance, if an organization experienced an accidental death when an individual served was strangled after slipping through guard rails on a bed, a videotape or photo of the bed with guard rails in place provides evidence of the position of the device following the event. The team should not rely on the memory of anyone. Instead, complete notes, audiotapes, videotapes, photographs, and drawings ensure accuracy and thoroughness of information collection. In addition, they aid in reporting the team's progress. See Sidebar 3-4, page 58, for ways of recording information.

In all cases, the team should seek guidance from the organization's legal counsel regarding protection of information from discovery through its inclusion in peer review and other means. The team should also seek guidance from the organization's ethics committee concerning patient confidentiality and the information collected during the root cause analysis (see Chapter 2, pages 33–34).

The team must ensure focus of information or data collection. Collecting a huge amount of information, much of which might not be related in any way, is both unproductive and confusing. To focus collection efforts, examine the problem statement and collect data along potential lines of inquiry. Figure 1-2, page 14, can provide guidance into potential lines of inquiry. For example, if the problem statement such as, "Patient

---

Sidebar 3-4. Ways to Record Information

The following media can be used to record information obtained during a root cause analysis:

· Written notes;
· Audiotapes;
· Photographs or drawings; and
· Videotapes.

It is important that the team obtains legal counsel on how to protect the information from discovery.

---

jumped from unsecured window," suggests an environment of care or human resources problem, then collect data relevant to training, security systems, and so forth. A sampling of information that might be collected relevant to the suicide, elopement, treatment delay, and medication examples described in Sidebar 3-1, pages 46–47, follows.

Information to be collected in the **suicide** investigation might include an environment of care inventory of all fixtures in the behavioral health care units, and data on which fixtures are "breakaway compliant" and which are not. That is, those that are or are not capable of breaking automatically in response to a predetermined external force (for example, the weight of an individual).

Information to be collected in the **elopement** investigation might include an environment of care inventory of unattended or unmonitored exits; availability and functionality of wander prevention technology, such as electric bracelets and "wired" exits; data related to the thoroughness and frequency of

initial resident assessment and ongoing reassessment for elopement risk; and information regarding how information about individuals at risk for elopement is integrated into initial and ongoing care plans.

Information to be collected in the **treatment delay** investigation might include data about how test results are processed within the organization and how staff is trained in these processes initially and on a continuing basis. Data related to competence assessment testing and staffing levels would also be valuable.

Information to be collected in the **medication error** investigation might include data on how medication orders are transmitted to local pharmacies and the percentage of queries and errors due to illegible physician handwriting, misinterpretation of physician handwriting, oral orders, and order transcription. Data related to the frequency of nurse communication about a new medication and patient education efforts would also be valuable.

While information or data collection occurs throughout the root cause analysis process, the team may also want to gather three key types of information at this early stage witness statements, physical evidence, and documentary evidence—as addressed below.

Witness Statements and Observations

Interviews with staff members can provide a wealth of information during a number of stages of root cause analysis. Closely following an event or near miss event, interviews with staff members *directly* involved can probe for what happened or almost happened and why (proximate causes). Interviews with staff members *indirectly* involved can explore possible root causes. Later in the process, interviews can provide insight into possible improvement initiatives and implementation strategies.

Conducting interviews is both an art and a science. Some people do it well; some do not. The team should carefully consider who is best suited to interview each subject and the best possible timing and sequence of interviews to be conducted. The goal of the interview is to determine facts, possible systemic causes, and identify improvement opportunities—*not* to place blame. The team should identify all likely interview candidates at each stage and be aware that people tend to forget information or remember it incorrectly, rationalize situations, and perceive situations differently.

Four discrete stages of what normally appears to be a continuous interview process are preparing for the interview, opening the interview, conducting the interview, and closing the interview.[6] The following descriptions are adapted from the book *The Root Cause Analysis Handbook*.

When *preparing for the interview*, the interviewer plans the interview. This involves reviewing previously collected information, developing carefully worded interview questions that are open-ended, scheduling the interview, determining how information will be recorded and documented, preparing to answer questions that the interviewee is likely to raise, identifying material that should be available as a reference during the interview, and establishing the physical setting. Carefully worded responses to such questions as, "Why do you want to talk with me?" and "What will you do with the information I provide?" can go a long way toward reducing the interviewee's defensiveness. So can a neutral setting where privacy is ensured and interruptions avoided.

When *opening the interview*, the interviewer should greet the interviewee, exchange informal conversation, state the purpose of the interview, and answer the interviewee's questions. The goal is to establish rapport, put the interviewee at ease, establish credibility, and get the interviewee involved in the interview process as quickly as possible. The

---

Tip: Overcoming Interviewee Defensiveness

- Restate the focus and purpose of the interview and reiterate that information obtained will be used to help prevent future occurrences of an adverse event, rather than to fix blame.
- Send positive, supportive messages through statements such as, "What you've said is so helpful," and "I understand, and you've obviously given this a lot of good thought."
- Gently ask about a defensive reaction and probe why the interviewee feels threatened (take great care here to ensure that this will not do more harm than good).

---

interviewer should indicate the amount of time required for the interview so that the interviewee knows what to expect.

When *conducting the interview*, the interviewer poses his or her open-ended questions. Open-ended questions elicit information by encouraging more than a yes or no response. In contrast, leading questions put words in the interviewee's mouth (for example, "This was only a minor problem, wasn't it?"). There are a number of different ways to pose such questions and use a variety of question types to ensure that the questions sound natural, several of which are shown in Sidebar 3-5, page 60. Keep in mind that the way questions are asked can often affect people's memories and their willingness to cooperate.

A two-step probing technique, using an exploratory question followed by a follow-up question asking "why," can yield valuable information (for example, the sequence of "What can you tell me about the administration of restraints in the unit?" followed by "Why do you think this is the case?"). This technique should be reserved for important areas because its repetition could make the interviewee feel "drilled."

Sidebar 3-5.
Types of Open-ended Questions

Open-ended questions ensure that the interviewee provides more than a simple yes or no answer. Three types of open-ended questions that can be used effectively to gain the depth and breadth of information needed during interviews follow:

Exploratory Questions

Exploratory questions can be used effectively to begin the discussion or a new topic. They encourage the interviewee to provide both comprehensive and in-depth information. Examples are

- "What can you tell me about ... ?"
- "What can you recall about ... ?"

Follow-up Questions

Often, it may be necessary to clarify or amplify information provided by the interviewee. Follow-up questions can help. Examples are

- "What do you mean by ... ?"
- "Can you tell me more about ... ?"
- "What is ... ?"
- "How did this come about?"

Comment Questions

Comment questions (or statements) encourage elaboration and express interest while not sounding like a question. Examples are

- "Can you tell me more about that?"
- "Could you please describe that further?"

Source: Adapted from Ammerman M: *The Root Cause Analysis Handbook: A Simplified Approach to Identifying, Correcting, and Reporting Workplace Errors*. New York: Quality Resources, 1998, pp 53–54.

Throughout the interview, the interviewer should listen well, avoid interrupting the subject, avoid being overtalkative, ask purposeful questions, and summarize to ensure a proper understanding of what the subject has related. The interviewer should also be aware of his or her own body language, as well as of the interviewee's body language and other nonverbal cues.

When *closing the interview*, the interviewer should check to ensure that he or she has obtained all necessary information, ask the interviewee if he or she has any questions or concerns, summarize the complete interview to ensure that the information accurately reflects the interviewee's words, and thank the interviewee, expressing appreciation for his or her time, honesty, and assistance.

After the interviewee leaves the interview area, the interviewer documents any further observations and identifies follow-up items. Conclusions and results are communicated to the root cause analysis team, as appropriate.

Group interviews can be more efficient than individual interviews, but disadvantages should be considered and weighed with care. Disadvantages include dominance by more vocal members of the group and the emergence of "group think," which can stifle individual accounts of an event.

When in-person interviews are not possible, telephone interviews can provide an alternative. However, the telephone has some serious limitations. It is much more difficult to establish and maintain rapport when eye contact is not part of the equation, and, of course, nonverbal cues are much harder to read. Written responses from an observer to specific questions raised by the team are another alternative (see Worksheet 3-6, pages 69–72). However, this means is less likely than either in-person or telephone interviews to elicit in-depth information. A matter as seemingly trivial as how much space is provided for answers on the form can have a significant impact on the quantity of information provided. In addition, when the observer must put something in writing, his or her concern about the privacy and confidentiality of the information may increase defensiveness, thereby preventing full disclosure and honesty.

So as not to alarm the interviewee, be sure to remind them that follow-up interviews are a routine part of the root cause analysis process and they do not necessarily imply suspicion.

Physical Evidence

Physical evidence related to the event or near miss should be gathered at an early stage. As described in Chapter 2, page 37, preserving the evidence immediately following the event or near miss can be essential to understanding why an event occurred or almost occurred. In many instances, physical evidence inadvertently (or deliberately) may be taken, misplaced, destroyed, moved, or altered in some way.

Interviews with personnel closest to the event can help the team identify relevant physical evidence, including equipment, materials, and devices. Physical evidence for a sentinel event involving a medication error, for example, might include the drug vial, syringe, prescription, IV drip, filter straws, and medication storage area. Physical evidence for a suicide in a 24-hour care setting might include breakaway bars and fixtures in the shower or elsewhere, a window, a ceiling, and other sites. Physical evidence for a wrong-site surgery might include the X rays, the operative arena, surgical instruments, and so forth.

The evidence should be thoroughly inspected by a knowledgeable team member, ad hoc member, or consultant. Perhaps equipment was not fully assembled or parts were missing. Observations from the inspection should be documented. All physical evidence should be labeled with information on the source, location, date and time collected, basic

content, and name of individual collecting it, and then secured in a separate area, if feasible. If not, such as with a large piece of equipment, the item should be tagged to indicate that it failed and that its use is prohibited, pending investigation results.

Documentary Evidence

Documentary evidence includes all material in paper or electronic format that is relevant to the event or possible event. This could include

- patient records, physician orders, medication profiles, laboratory test results, and all other documents used to record patient status and care;
- policies and procedures, correspondence, and meeting minutes;
- human resources–related documents such as performance evaluations, competence assessments, and physician profiles;
- indicator data used to measure performance; and
- maintenance information such as work orders, equipment logs, instructions for use, vendor manuals, and testing and inspection records.

All such evidence should be examined, secured, and labeled appropriately.

Documentary evidence will vary considerably, based on the actual sentinel event or possible sentinel event. Examples of documentary evidence for various error types follow. This information is a starting place in considering the kind of documentary evidence needed for any organization's root cause analysis.

For a **medication error** involving the administration of the wrong medication and the subsequent death of a patient, documentary evidence could include

- the patient's medical record;
- trending data on medication errors;
- procedures for drug-allergy interaction checking;
- pharmacy lot number logs;
- pharmacy recall procedure;
- maintenance logs for equipment repair;
- downtime logs for computer software;

- equipment procedure logs for mixing of solutions;
- the error report to the U.S. Pharmacopoeia and state licensing agency;
- lab test results of drug samples; and
- interdepartmental and interorganizational memos or reports regarding the event.

For a **mechanical error** involving the shutoff of oxygen and the subsequent death of a patient, documentary evidence could include

- procedures for informing patient care areas of downtime of mechanical or life support systems;
- construction and technical documents and drawings of medical gas distribution system;
- inspection, performance measurement, and testing policies and procedures;
- policies and procedures for shutoff of utility systems;
- utility system performance measurement data;
- documents related to utility systems planning process;
- management competence assessment programs;
- technical staff training, retraining, and competence assessment programs in utilities systems processes;
- incident and emergency reporting procedures; and
- maintenance procedures and logs.

For a **patient suicide**, documentary evidence could include

- the patient's history and physical on admission;
- staff observation notes;
- attendance logs for unit activities;
- policies and procedures for patient observation;
- an inventory of items in the patient's possession on admission;
- the patient's psychosocial assessment; and
- all physician and nursing notes prior to the incident.

Literature Review

At this point and throughout the root cause analysis, a thorough review of the professional literature is an important component of the root cause analysis process. Literature searches can yield helpful information about the event at hand and other organizations' experiences with a similar event. Literature can help identify possible root causes and improvement strategies. Appropriate associations and societies can provide a good starting point in the review process. Obtain a variety of information on the subject. A review of other organizations' practices and experiences can help avoid mistakes and inspire creative thinking. Information that might be obtained to investigate causes and improvement strategies for the example sentinel events includes the following.

For the **suicide** event, the team might obtain suicide risk assessment policies, procedures, and forms from other organizations. A team member might conduct an online literature search to obtain suicide risk assessment protocols from relevant professional journals.

For the **elopement** event, the team might obtain resident assessment policies, procedures, and forms from other long term care organizations and specifically, information related to how they assess at-risk-for-elopement status. The facility or safety manager might obtain information from other organizations related to systems used to ensure appropriate security in the environment of care, such as wander prevention technology. Assessment protocols from relevant professional journals might be helpful as well.

For the **treatment delay** event, the team might obtain policies, procedures, and protocols for communicating abnormal test findings from the professional literature and peer ambulatory care organizations. Training and competence assessment literature could also provide insight for improvement strategies. Professional organizations might be a source of information on criteria for calling in additional specialists.

For the **medication error** event, the team might contact other home care organizations to obtain information about the policies and protocols used to ensure a safe medication use process. An online literature review could provide improvement strategies recommended by other health care organizations following a sentinel event or near miss.

Tools to Use

The team should begin to consider performance measurement tools that might be helpful in the next step of the root cause analysis—searching for proximate causes and determining what happened and why. Information can be collected on such tools as brainstorming, flowcharts, cause-and-effect diagrams, Pareto charts, scatter diagrams, affinity diagrams, bar graphs, line graphs, pie graphs, Gantt charts, and time lines.

 Tools: *Brainstorming, flowcharts, cause-and-effect diagrams, Pareto charts, scatter diagrams, affinity diagrams, bar graphs, line graphs, pie graphs, Gantt charts, time lines*

References

1. Phillips KM: *The Power of Health Care Teams: Strategies for Success*. Oakbrook Terrace, IL: Joint Commission on Accreditation of Healthcare Organizations, 1997, pp 18, 30.
2. Nelson EC, Batalden PB, Ryer JC (eds): *Clinical Improvement Action Guide*. Oakbrook Terrace, IL: Joint Commission Resources, 1998, p 27.
3. Phillips, p 43.
4. Wilson PF, Dell LD, Anderson GF: *Root Cause Analysis: A Tool for Total Quality Management*. Milwaukee: ASQC Quality Press, 1993, pp 39, 40.
5. Nelson et al, pp 34–35.
6. Ammerman M: *The Root Cause Analysis Handbook: A Simplified Approach to Identifying, Correcting, and Reporting Workplace Errors*. New York: Quality Resources, 1998, pp 49–61.

Worksheet 3-1. Composing the Team

Fill in the team leader, facilitator (if necessary), and team members, including ad hoc members who serve on an "as needed" basis. Ensure interdisciplinary representation by including information such as job titles, degrees, and responsibilities.

Core Team Members

1. Leader _____

2. Facilitator _____

3. _____

4. _____

5. _____

6. _____

7. _____

8. _____

9. _____

10. _____

Ad Hoc Members

_____

_____

_____

_____

_____

_____

_____

Worksheet 3-2. Defining the Problem

Use this space to formulate a simple, one-sentence definition of the event or near miss.

A sentinel event occurred: What happened?

_____

_____

_____

_____

_____

_____

_____

_____

A near miss occurred: What nearly happened?

_____

_____

_____

_____

_____

_____

_____

_____

_____

Worksheet 3-3. Identifying Risk-Prone Systems

Use this worksheet to identify risk-prone systems within your organization.

Systems involving variable input include

_____

_____

Complex systems include

_____

_____

Nonstandardized systems include

_____

_____

Tightly coupled systems include

_____

_____

Systems with tight time constraints include

_____

_____

Systems with a hierarchical, nonteam structure include

_____

_____

Worksheet 3-4. Sharpening an Aim Statement

1. The organization's aim is to improve the quality and value of (fill in the name of the care process):

   _____

   _____

   _____

   _____.

2. This process starts with _____

   _____

   and ends when_____

   _____.

3. By working on this process, the team expects that (fill in the anticipated better and measurable outcomes)

   _____

   _____

   _____

   _____.

4. It is important to work on this process now because (insert reasons that make this important)

   _____

   _____

   _____

   _____.

Worksheet 3-5. Preliminary Planning

Overall strategy

☐ Does it include the team's aim?   ☐ Is it objective?   ☐ Is it measurable?

Key steps/initiatives	Individual responsible	Target date
_____	_____	_____
_____	_____	_____
_____	_____	_____
_____	_____	_____
_____	_____	_____
_____	_____	_____
_____	_____	_____

Reporting mechanisms
Who receives copies of the reports?

_____

_____

_____

_____

_____

Are the reports or other output from the team

☐ Informative?   ☐ Accurate?   ☐ Timely?

Worksheet 3-6. Gathering Information

Use this worksheet as a place to start in gathering written information from individuals who cannot be interviewed in person or by telephone. Be aware that the amount of space you provide under each question will often determine the amount of information provided by the respondent. If a detailed answer to a certain question is desired, be sure to leave plenty of space and provide a prompt such as, "Please provide as much information as possible."

What conditions existed prior to the event?

_____

_____

_____

_____

_____

_____

What procedures or processes were being conducted prior to and during the event?

_____

_____

_____

_____

_____

_____

Worksheet 3-6. Gathering Information (continued)

Who was present and involved in the event?

_____

_____

_____

_____

_____

_____

What indicated that a problem was occurring?

_____

_____

_____

_____

_____

_____

_____

How did you respond?

_____

_____

_____

_____

_____

_____

Worksheet 3-6. Gathering Information (continued)

How did others in the area respond?

_____

_____

_____

_____

_____

_____

_____

What procedures or processes might have been associated with the event?

_____

_____

_____

_____

_____

_____

_____

What might have caused the event?

_____

_____

_____

_____

_____

_____

_____

Worksheet 3-6. Gathering Information (continued)

How might the event be prevented in the future?

_____

_____

_____

_____

_____

_____

_____

_____

_____

Any other comments or thoughts?

_____

_____

_____

_____

_____

_____

_____

_____

_____

_____

Chapter 4

Determining What Happened and Why: The Search for Proximate Causes

Step 1: Organize a Team
Step 2: Define the Problem
Step 3: Study the Problem
Step 4: Determine What Happened
Step 5: Identify Contributing Process Factors
Step 6: Identify Other Contributing Factors
Step 7: Measure—Collect and Assess Data on Proximate and Underlying Causes
Step 8: Design and Implement Interim Changes
Step 9: Identify Which Systems Are Involved—The Root Causes
Step 10: Prune the List of Root Causes
Step 11: Confirm Root Causes and Consider Their Interrelationships
Step 12: Explore and Identify Risk Reduction Strategies
Step 13: Formulate Improvement Actions
Step 14: Evaluate Proposed Improvement Actions
Step 15: Design Improvements
Step 16: Ensure Acceptability of the Action Plan
Step 17: Implement the Improvement Plan
Step 18: Develop Measures of Effectiveness and Ensure Their Success
Step 19: Evaluate Implementation of Improvement Efforts
Step 20: Take Additional Action
Step 21: Communicate the Results

This chapter provides guidance on how a team can search for proximate or direct causes. It represents the first level of probing to determine in more detail what happened, or nearly happened, and why. The team must also look at process and other contributing factors. This chapter also provides information on choosing what to measure and analyze further so that the team can determine root causes and an effective improvement plan. Figure 1-3, pages 18–20, from Chapter 1, provides the framework for this and subsequent steps of root cause analysis.

4

Step Four: Determine What Happened

Prior to this point in the process, the team has created a very simple, one-sentence definition of what happened or could have happened. The next step involves creating a more detailed description or definition of the event. The description provides the *when*, *where*, and *how* details of the event. The definition should include

- a brief description of what happened;
- mention of where and when the event occurred (place, date, day of week, and time); and
- identification of the area or services affected by the event.

For example, with a sentinel event involving "the death of an individual served in restraints," a more detailed definition of the event might state, "Death of an

18-year old male from burns and smoke inhalation following a fire started by the individual with matches in a room in Unit E where the individual was restrained. Event occurred on Friday, January 1, at 11 AM." The relevant areas for this sentinel event might be nursing, medicine, security, and physical plant. See Worksheet 4-1, page 83, for questions to ask in developing a detailed definition of the event.

In creating this more detailed definition of the event, team members should be careful not to jump to conclusions concerning what happened prior to completing the root cause analysis. For example, perhaps the team's problem statement at this point reads, "80-year-old female found in room beside her bed, lying on floor dead. Event occurred sometime between 0200 and 0330, Thursday, March 4." Did the individual die because of the fall? Or, did the individual fall after or while dying? A root cause analysis will help the team identify the cause of death. In this example, relevant areas or services affected by the event might include nursing (to investigate monitoring systems and medication administration), biomedical (to investigate the type of bed, alarm, and call light system), staffing office (to investigate whether the type of staff—regular or float—impacted the event), education (to investigate orientation and training provided to staff and patient), pharmacy (to investigate patient medications), and medical staff protocols (to investigate medications ordered for the patient).

It is often helpful to determine the sequence of events by developing a time line or flowchart. These tools can help the team retain focus on the facts of the event. Ensure that the source of each fact is noted on the tool so the source can be consulted if more information is needed.

Tools: *Flowchart, time line*

Step Five: Identify Contributing Process Factors

5

Root cause analysis involves repeatedly asking "Why?" in order to identify the underlying root causes of an event or possible event. At this point, the team asks the first of a series of "why" questions. The goal of the first "why" question is to identify the proximate causes of the event. *Proximate* or *direct causes* are those most apparent or immediate reasons for an event. They involve factors lying closest to the origin of an event, and they generally can be gleaned by asking, "Why did the event happen?" As mentioned in Chapter 1 (pages 6–8), a proximate cause typically involves a special-cause variation. Special-cause variation is not inherently present in the process. It is intermittent and unpredictable. If the team is measuring a process using a control chart, special-cause variation will appear as those points outside the control limits. In contrast, common-cause variation will appear as points between the control limits.

Tool: *Control chart*

In most cases, identifying the proximate causes will be simple; in other cases, it might take some digging. For example, in the restraint-related death, proximate or direct causes could include "missed observation" and "patient possessed contraband matches." In the case of the patient found dead by her bed, proximate causes could include "failure to monitor patient," "bed alarm not working," "call light not working," "patient not properly oriented to use of call light," "incorrect sedation dispensed," or "incorrect administration of sedation."

Underlying causes of proximate causes in the health care environment may relate to the provision of care or to other processes. Hence, identification of the patient care processes or activities involved in the sentinel event or potential sentinel event will help the team identify contributing causes. At this point, asking and answering these three questions will assist the team:

1. Which processes were involved in the event, or almost led to an event?
2. What are the steps, and linkages between the steps, in the process, as designed, as routinely performed, and as occurred with the sentinel event?
3. Which steps and linkages were involved in, or contributed to, the event?

A variety of tools can help ensure a thorough response to these questions. A flowchart is a useful way to visualize the response to "What are the steps in the process?" Brainstorming can also be used to identify processes and supplement the list of process steps to ensure that all relevant steps are included. Cause-and-effect diagrams, change analysis, and failure mode and effects analysis (FMEA) are useful techniques in analyzing the response to "Which steps and linkages were involved in, or contributed to, the event?"

Tools: *Brainstorming, flowchart, cause-and-effect diagram, change analysis, failure mode and effects analysis (FMEA)*

The team can then probe further by asking three more questions:

1. What is currently done to prevent failure at this step or its link with the next step?
2. What is currently done to protect against a bad outcome if there is failure at this step or linkage?
3. What other areas or services are affected?

Comparing the flowchart of the process as designed and specified in written policies and procedures to the flowcharts of the process as routinely performed or as occurring with the sentinel event can alert the team to staff actions that circumvent policies and procedures either knowingly or unknowingly.

Fault tree analysis can also be used to study current failure prevention activities. Barrier analysis can be helpful in looking at what is currently done to protect against a bad outcome if there is a failure. FMEA can

be a useful tool in examining other affected areas or services. Use Worksheet 4-2, page 84, as a summary of questions to raise and tools to consider using.

Tools: *Fault tree analysis, barrier analysis, failure mode and effects analysis (FMEA)*

6 Step Six: Identify Other Contributing Factors

In the health care environment, proximate causes tend to fall into a number of distinct categories beyond, and in addition to, process factors. These include

- human factors;
- equipment factors;
- controllable or uncontrollable environmental factors; and
- other factors.

To identify the proximate cause of an event involving human factors, the team might ask, "What human factors were relevant to the outcome?"

To identify the proximate cause of an event involving equipment factors, the team might ask, "How did the equipment performance affect the outcome?"

To identify the proximate cause of an event involving environmental factors, the team might ask, "What factors directly affected the outcome? Were such factors within or truly beyond the organization's control?"

Finally, the team might ask, "Are there any other factors that have directly influenced this outcome?" Figures 4-1 through 4-3, pages 76–77, identify common factors associated with procedure-, training-, and equipment-related failures. Use Worksheet 4-3, pages 85–86, to identify factors closest to the event.

Continuing the example involving the death of an individual served in restraints following a fire, the team might conclude that proximate causes included

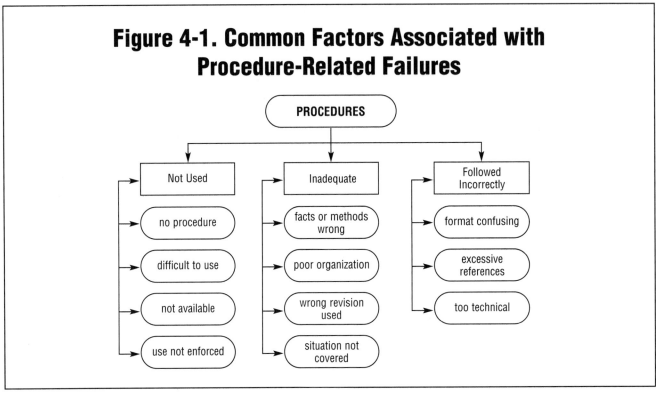

Source: Mobley RK: *Root Cause Failure Analysis*. Boston: Newnes, 1999, p 40. Used with permission.

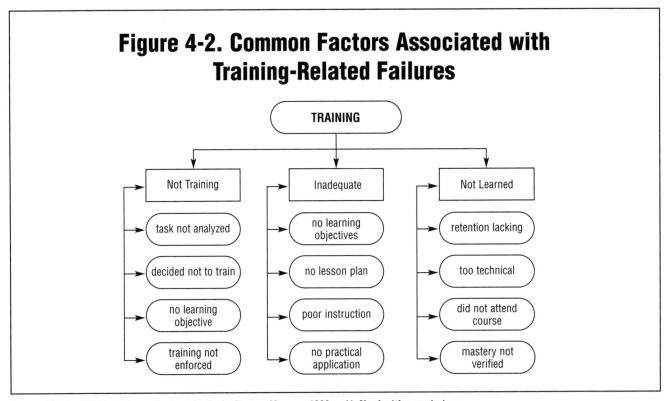

Source: Mobley RK: *Root Cause Failure Analysis*. Boston: Newnes, 1999, p 41. Used with permission.

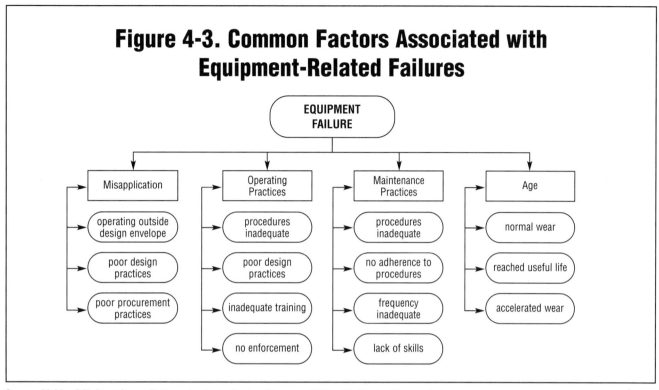

Figure 4-3. Common Factors Associated with Equipment-Related Failures

Source: Mobley RK: *Root Cause Failure Analysis*. Boston: Newnes, 1999, p 38. Used with permission.

- human factors involving failure to follow observation procedures, failure to implement contraband checking procedures, an lack of de-escalation training;
- assessment factors involving failure of the safety or patient assessment tools, incomplete patient assessment, assessment beyond the scope of staff (for example, completed in the emergency department by staff with no behavioral health assessment competence);
- environmental factors involving difficulty in conducting regular patient observations due to the design of space; and
- controllable equipment factors involving failure of smoke detector.

Similarly, in identifying the proximate causes for a suicide, a team might conclude that proximate causes include

- human factors involving failure to follow policies on precaution orders or failure to conduct appropriate staff education/training;

- assessment process factors involving a faulty initial assessment process that did not include identification of past history of suicide attempts or an immediate psychiatric consultation;
- process or human factors involving a faulty history and physical assessment that did not identify patient suicide risk factors; and
- equipment factors involving a nonfunctional paging system that delayed communication with the individual's physician.

Brainstorming to identify all possible or potential contributing causes may be a useful technique for teams at this stage of the root cause analysis. Following traditional brainstorming ground rules, such as "there is no bad idea," and ensuring that team members do not express reactions or provide commentary as ideas are expressed, are critical to success. The focus must be on improving patient outcomes rather than individual performance. Affinity diagrams can be used to help sort or organize the causes or potential causes into natural, related groupings. Cause-and-effect diagrams can help to highlight the numerous factors involved in the event.

Tools: *Brainstorming, affinity diagram, cause-and-effect diagram*

While asking questions to uncover causes, the team leader will want to keep team members focused on processes, not people. By repeatedly asking "Why?" the team can continue working until it feels it has exhausted all possible questions and causes. The importance of this stage cannot be overstated. It provides the initial substance for the root cause analysis without which a team cannot proceed.

After sorting and analyzing the cause list, the team may begin determining which process or system each cause is a part of and whether the cause is a special or common cause in that process or system. This process, described fully in the next chapter, helps to unearth system-based root causes.

 7

Step Seven: Measure—Collect and Assess Data on Proximate and Underlying Causes

To advance further toward discovering root causes, the team must explore in depth proximate and underlying causes. This exploration involves measurement—collecting and assessing relevant data. While this exploration is presented here as step 7, data collection and analysis initiatives may occur throughout root cause analysis and need not necessarily be sequential or follow step 6 and precede step 8.

Measurement is the process of collecting and aggregating data. The process helps assess the level of performance, determine whether improvement actions are necessary, and ascertain whether improvement has occurred.

The first purpose of measurement is to provide a baseline when little objective evidence exists about a process. For example, a health care organization may

want to learn more about the current level of staff competence. A dementia long term care or psychiatric special care unit may want to know more about the effectiveness of the bed alarm systems to prevent patient falls and elopement. Specific indicators for a particular outcome or a particular step in a process may be used for ongoing data collection. Once assessed, these data can help management and staff determine whether a process is ineffective and needs more intensive analysis. Data about costs, including costs of faulty or ineffective processes, may also be of significant interest to leaders and can be part of ongoing performance measurement.

The second purpose of measurement, more the focus here, is to gain more information about a process chosen for assessment and improvement. For example, perhaps a performance rate varies significantly from the previous year, from shift to shift, or from the statistical average. A team may be measuring staff compliance with the organization's restraint policy, for instance. Records may indicate that the staff on duty during weekend hours did not properly document the monitoring of individuals in restraint or obtain appropriate orders for restraint use. Or, perhaps the data indicate that restraints are used with an increased frequency when specific personnel are present. Perhaps monitoring problems or inappropriate restraint use is suspected as part of a root cause of a sentinel event. Such findings may cause a health care organization to focus on a given process to determine opportunities for improvement. The target for further study is usually time limited and can test a specific population, a specific diagnosis, a specific service provided, or an organization management issue. Detailed measurement would then be necessary to gather data about exactly how the process performs and about factors affecting that performance.

The third purpose of measurement is to determine the effectiveness of improvement actions. For example, a nursing unit that begins to use a new piece of equipment will need to establish a baseline performance rate and continue to measure use. Measurement can also demonstrate that key processes (for example, the preparation and administration of medications) are in control. Once a process has been stabilized at an acceptable level of performance, it may be measured periodically to verify that the improvement has been sustained. Measurement to monitor improvement actions is described fully in Chapter 6 (pages 122–123).

In summary, data are collected to monitor the stability of existing processes, identify opportunities for improvement, identify changes that will lead to improvement, and maintain changes.

Choosing what to measure is absolutely critical at all stages of root cause analysis—in probing for root causes and in assessing whether a recommended change or action represents an actual improvement (see Sidebar 4-1 right). Measurement requires indicators that are stable, consistent, understandable, easy to use, and reliable. *Indicators* or *performance measures* are devices or tools for quantifying the level of performance that actually occurs. They are valid if they identify events that merit review and they are reliable if they accurately and completely identify occurrences (see Sidebar 4-2 bottom right).

Examples of an outcome indicator are "catheter-related sepsis for patients with a central venous access device" or "percentage of patients at risk for falls who actually experience falls while in the health care organization." An example of a process indicator is "patients over 65 years of age having medication monitoring for drugs that can decrease renal function."

The two broadest types of indicators are sentinel event indicators and aggregate data indicators. A *sentinel event indicator* identifies an individual event or phenomenon that is significant enough to trigger further investigation each time it occurs. Such indicators are well known in risk management. They help ensure that each event is promptly evaluated to

---

Sidebar 4-1.
Choosing What to Measure

Choosing what to measure is extremely important. An organization may wish to start by defining the broad processes or systems most likely to underlie proximate causes. For example, if a team is investigating a medication error involving the process used to communicate an order to the pharmacy and the process used by pharmacy staff to check the dosage ordered, the team may decide to measure the following for a defined period of time:

- Time elapsed between when an order is written by medical staff and when the pharmacy receives the order by fax, pickup, or phone;
- Time elapsed between when the dosage is checked by pharmacy staff and when the medication is dispensed; and
- Time elapsed between when the medication is dispensed and when the medication is administered.

Sidebar 4-2. Definition of an Indicator or Measure

An indicator (or measure) is
- quantitative—it is expressed in units of measurement;
- valid—it identifies events that merit review;
- reliable—it accurately and completely identifies occurrences; and
- a measure of a process or outcome—it involves a goal-directed series of activities or the results of performance.

prevent future occurrences. As required by Joint Commission performance improvement requirements, all health care organizations must monitor the performance of processes that involve risks or may result in sentinel events.

Although sentinel event indicators are useful to ensure patient safety, they are less useful in measuring the overall level of performance in an organization. In contrast, an *aggregate data indicator* quantifies a process or outcome related to many cases. Unlike a sentinel event, an event identified by an aggregate data indicator may occur frequently. Aggregate data indicators are divided into two groups, rate-based indicators and continuous variable indicators.

Rate-Based Indicators

Rate-based indicators express the proportion of the number of occurrences to the entire group within which the occurrence could take place, as in the following examples:

$$\frac{\text{Patients receiving cesarean sections}}{\text{All patients who deliver}}$$

$$\frac{\text{Total number of elopements}}{\substack{\text{Patients at risk for elopement} \\ \text{(wandering and confused)}}}$$

$$\frac{\text{Patients with central line catheter infections}}{\text{All patients with central line access devices}}$$

$$\frac{\text{Patient falls associated with adverse drug reactions}}{\text{All patient falls}}$$

The rate can also express a ratio comparing the occurrences identified with a different, but related phenomenon. For example:

$$\frac{\text{Patients with central line infections}}{\text{Central line days}}$$

Continuous Variable Indicators

This type of aggregate data indicator measures performance along a continuous scale. For example, a continuous variable indicator might show the precise weight in kilograms of an individual receiving total parenteral nutrition (TPN). Or, it might record the

number of written pharmacist recommendations accepted by the attending physicians. While a rate-based indicator might relate the number of patients approaching goal weights to total number of patients on TPN, a continuous variable indicator would measure the patient's average weight change (that is, the patient's weight in one month minus the patient's weight the previous month).

See Checklist 4-1, page 81, for criteria that will help the team ensure that the measure or indicator selected will actually be appropriate for monitoring performance. See Sidebar 4-3, page 81, for key questions the team should ask about measurement throughout the root cause analysis process.

Additional information on measurement, including how to measure the effectiveness of improvement initiatives and assure the success of measurement, appears in Chapter 6 (pages 122–123).

8 Step Eight: Design and Implement Interim Changes

Even at this early stage, when the team has identified only proximate causes, some quick or immediate "fixes" may be appropriate. For example, in the case of an organization that experienced the suicide of an individual served who was not identified as being at risk for suicide, the organization could immediately evaluate its current risk assessment tool to learn whether it meets current standards of practice. Or, still, it could start conducting mandatory in-service training for all staff on suicide risk assessment. Or the organization could place all patients with psychiatric or substance abuse diagnoses on suicide precautions. Or, rather, the organization could address environment of care issues such as nonbreakaway showerheads and bed linens. In addition, the organization could evaluate the suicide risk assessment tool and the process used to check for contraband, and initiate meetings with the medical staff to discuss revisions to requirements for histories and physicals. A Gantt chart used by one organization

Checklist 4-1. Criteria to Ensure Appropriate Data Collection

Choosing what to measure is critical. So is ensuring that the data collected are appropriate to the desired measurement. The following checklist includes criteria to help the team ensure that the data collected are appropriate for monitoring performance:

☐ The measure can identify the events it was intended to identify.

☐ The measure has a documented numerator and has a denominator statement or description of the population to which the measure is applicable.

☐ The measure has defined data elements and allowable values.

☐ The measure can detect changes in performance over time.

☐ The measure allows for comparison over time within the organization or between the organization and other entities.

☐ The data intended for collection are available.

☐ Results can be reported in a way that is useful to the organization and other interested customers.

Sidebar 4-3. Key Questions About Measurement

Throughout the root cause analysis, the team should ask the following questions concerning measurement:

• What will be measured? (This defines what is critical to determining root causes.)

• Why will this be measured? (This verifies the criticality of what will be measured.)

• What does the organization hope to gain from such measurement? (This describes the incentives of measurement.)

• Who will perform the measurement?

• How frequently is the measuring?

• How will the data be used when the measurement is completed?

• Is the measure or measurement reliable?

• Is the measurement a one-time event or periodic process?

• What resources are needed for the measurement? What are available?

• Do the measures consider dimensions of performance?

to outline the key steps and time frames for a plan to eliminate proximate causes that led to a patient suicide appears as Figure 4-4, page 82.

 Tool: *Gantt chart*

In the case of an organization that experienced a wrong-site surgery, the organization could require a second staff member to observe operating room team procedures to identify processes not in place or not being followed.

Teams conducting root cause analysis need not wait until they finish their analysis to begin designing and implementing changes. During the process of asking "Why?" potential interventions emerge. Intermediate changes may not only be appropriate but necessary. First, they may be needed to reduce an immediate risk. For example, an unsecured window may need to be repaired and secured; an intoxicated employee should be removed from the environment immediately; and broken or malfunctioning equipment should be removed from the area of care, treatment, or service, and secured. Second, they may also uncover additional causes that were previously masked, but are critical to the search for the root cause. Finally, intermediate changes can be part of a plan-do-study-act (PDSA) cycle to test process redesign before implementing it

Figure 4-4. Proximate Causes of a Patient Suicide

ACTIVITY	3rd Qtr 2001			4th Qtr 2001			1st Qtr 2002			2nd Qtr 2002		
	Jul	Aug	Sep	Oct	Nov	Dec	Jan	Feb	Mar	Apr	May	Jun
Establish review team												
Expanded security rounds to include helipad												
Revised Suicide Precaution Policy												
Staff training: Suicide Precaution Policy												
Staff training: Assessment and interventions for patients with mental health needs												
Staff training: Patients leaving unit unattended												
Team meetings to assess plan-do-study-act (PDSA)												
Medical record review of all suicide precaution charts												
Concurrent assessment of patients on suicide precautions												

organizationwide. For instance, an organization may wish to test the use of new bathroom hardware in one room before changing hardware organizationwide.

The process of sorting through causes for the root cause has been called "identifying the web of causation." "The key point is to identify the web of causation and to intervene on as many levels as possible in this web. It is important to recognize that the deeper one progresses in the chain or web of causation, the closer one gets to underlying, structural (root) causes."[1] Hence, although the team may make intermediate improvements along the way, it should not stop the root cause analysis process before the root cause is identified and corrective action is taken. Where intermediate actions are planned, the team should identify

- *who* is responsible for implementation;
- *when* the actions will be implemented—including any pilot testing; and
- *how* the effectiveness of the actions will be evaluated.

Again, however worthy short-term solutions may be, the organization must not stop after implementing these, but rather continue probing more deeply to arrive at the root causes and possible long-term solutions. Chapter 5 addresses how the team can continue this effort.

Reference

1. Altman DG: Strategies for community health intervention: Promises, paradoxes, pitfalls. *Psychosom Med* 57(3):226–233, 1995.

Worksheet 4-1. Further Defining What Happened

In developing a more detailed definition of what happened, the team should consider the following three questions:

1. What are the details of the event? Write a brief, two- or three-sentence description.

_____

_____

_____

_____

_____

_____

2. When and where did the event occur (place, date, day of week, and time)?

_____

_____

_____

_____

_____

_____

3. What area(s) or service(s) was impacted?

_____

_____

_____

_____

_____

_____

Worksheet 4-2. Identifying Proximate Causes

To determine proximate causes of a sentinel event or possible sentinel event involving patient care or organization processes, the team can ask the following questions and consider using the following tools to aid in answering each question:

1. Which processes were involved or could have been involved in the event or near event?
    Tools: ☐ Brainstorming   ☐ Cause-and-effect diagram

    _____

    _____

2. What are the steps in the process, as designed?
    Tools: ☐ Flowchart   ☐ Brainstorming

    _____

    _____

3. Which steps were (or could have been) involved in, or contributed to, the event or near event?
    Tools: ☐ Cause-and-effect diagram   ☐ Change analysis ☐ Failure mode and effects analysis

    _____

    _____

4. What is currently done to prevent failure at this step?
    Tools: ☐ Fault tree analysis   ☐ Flowchart

    _____

    _____

5. What is currently done to protect against a negative outcome if there is failure at this step?
    Tool: ☐ Barrier analysis

    _____

    _____

6. What other areas or services are affected?
    Tools: ☐ Failure mode and effects analysis   ☐ Brainstorming

    _____

    _____

Worksheet 4-3. Identifying Factors Close to the Event

Use this worksheet to identify factors closest to the event or possible event.

Human factors included or could include

_____

_____

_____

_____

_____

_____

Equipment factors included or could include

_____

_____

_____

_____

_____

_____

Controllable environmental factors included or could include

_____

_____

_____

_____

_____

_____

Worksheet 4-3. Identifying Factors Close to the Event (continued)

Uncontrollable environmental factors included or could include

_____

_____

_____

_____

_____

_____

Other factors included or could include

_____

_____

_____

_____

_____

_____

Chapter 5

Identifying Root Causes

This chapter addresses how the team identifies and validates the root causes of a sentinel event or near miss sentinel event. This represents a deeper level of digging to determine the systemic roots of a problem. Root causes are the most fundamental causal factors of an event. As such, their origin lies in common-cause variation of organization systems. (A discussion of variation can be found in Chapter 1, pages 6–8.) Getting to the root cause of a sentinel event or near miss sentinel event takes a lot of time and effort. It involves asking "Why?" at least three to five times and then exploring the ramifications of each response. This chapter provides guidance on how to conduct such an exploration. Again, Figure 1-3, pages 18–20, in Chapter 1 provides the framework for this and subsequent steps of the root cause analysis.

Step 1: Organize a Team
Step 2: Define the Problem
Step 3: Study the Problem
Step 4: Determine What Happened
Step 5: Identify Contributing Process Factors
Step 6: Identify Other Contributing Factors
Step 7: Measure—Collect and Assess Data on Proximate and Underlying Causes
Step 8: Design and Implement Interim Changes
Step 9: Identify Which Systems Are Involved— The Root Causes
Step 10: Prune the List of Root Causes
Step 11: Confirm Root Causes and Consider Their Interrelationships
Step 12: Explore and Identify Risk Reduction Strategies
Step 13: Formulate Improvement Actions
Step 14: Evaluate Proposed Improvement Actions
Step 15: Design Improvements
Step 16: Ensure Acceptability of the Action Plan
Step 17: Implement the Improvement Plan
Step 18: Develop Measures of Effectiveness and Ensure Their Success
Step 19: Evaluate Implementation of Improvement Efforts
Step 20: Take Additional Action
Step 21: Communicate the Results

9 Step Nine: Identify Which Systems Are Involved—The Root Causes

The probing continues. At this point, the team has a detailed description of the event or near miss event and a list of proximate causes that describe the patient care processes and other factors that might have caused or contributed to the problem, or could do so in the future. The team has probably also started to collect data on proximate causes. Now the team again asks, "Why? Why did that proximate cause happen? What systems and processes underlie proximate factors?" The goal of asking questions at this stage is to identify the underlying causes for the proximate causes. For example, in the case of the elderly individual found dead on the floor by her bed, questions might include the following:

- Why was the patient not monitored for an hour to an hour and a half?
- Why was a new graduate nurse assigned to this patient's care? Did the nurse have the assistance of ancillary staff?
- How much orientation had the nurse completed?
- Why was the individual given a sedative?
- Why was the call light not by the individual's hand?

As in all stages of the process, it is critical to keep the team focused on probing for system or common-cause problems, rather than focusing on human errors. Teams often have trouble at this stage of the root cause analysis. The tendency is to stop short after identifying proximate causes and not to probe deeper. The probing must continue until a reason underlying a cause can no longer be identified. This, then, is a root cause.

Underlying causes may involve special-cause variation, common-cause variation, or both. Being special or common is not an inherent characteristic of the cause itself. Rather, it describes the relationship of the cause to a specific process or system. It is possible for the same cause to be a special cause in one process and a common cause in another. A flowchart of the process(es) at this stage may be very helpful.

Tool: *Flowchart*

For a special cause in a process, teams should search for the common cause in the system of which the process is a part. It is the larger system and its managers, not the process or process owners, that will need to be responsible for the redesigns that will reduce the likelihood of future sentinel events. Again, in most cases, a special cause of variation in one process is often found to be the result of, or permitted by, a common cause of variation in a larger system of which the process is a part. Identifying a special cause is only an initial step in a full evaluation.

> ### Tip: Clarify All Issues
>
> It is critical at this point for the team to clearly define the issues regarding the sentinel event and to be sure that team members share a common understanding of the issues. No matter how obvious the issues may seem, individual team members may not understand them in the same way.
>
> For example, a staff member may not consider identification of the surgical site by *all* operating room team members to be worth the time involved. Or, if a patient suffers a burn during surgery, surgical team members may not agree about whether the burn could have been affected by the proximity of the oxygen cannula to the cautery or how the cannula was handled during the cauterizing procedure.

For example, a special cause is created when one group of surgeons and their assistants do not follow hospital procedures for hand washing and this results in a sentinel event. This special cause might be part of a common-cause variation in a larger system: The hospital experiences high rates of postoperative infections resulting from insufficient education in sterile techniques and hand washing. Use Worksheet 5-1, page 98, to organize the team's probe for underlying causes.

Sentinel events and near misses can be very complex and involve multiple causes. Understanding causes is essential if the organization is to create lasting improvements. Certain tools can be particularly helpful in systematically looking at an event to determine its causes. Such tools include flowcharts, cause-and-effect diagrams, barrier analysis, failure mode and effects analysis, and fault tree analysis. The tools are designed to help root cause analysis team members understand processes and factors that contribute to both good and problematic performance. They are also designed to be used by any group studying a process. None of the tools requires a statistical background. They may be used singly or in combination to show the relationship between processes and factors, reach conclusions, and systematically analyze causes.

 Tools: *Flowchart, cause-and-effect diagram, barrier analysis, failure mode and effects analysis, fault tree analysis*

Cause-and-effect diagrams or fishbone diagrams are particularly helpful in categorizing and visualizing multiple system or process problems that have contributed to a sentinel event or near miss. The standard major categories coming off the main "spine" include people, procedures, equipment or materials, environment, and policies. Such categories as communication, education, leadership, and culture may also be appropriate. Subcauses branch off each major category.

Listing and categorizing the possible causal factors represent a logical starting point in the team's effort to determine the systems involved with the event or near miss. Common or root causes of a sentinel event in a health care organization can be categorized according to the important organization functions or processes performed by the organization. These include processes for
- human resources;
- information management;
- environmental management; and
- leadership—embracing corporate culture, encouragement of communication, and clear communication of priorities.

In addition, factors beyond an organization's control should be considered as a separate category. Organizations must exercise caution in assigning factors to this category, however. Although a causative factor may be beyond an organization's control, the *protection* of patients from the effects of the "uncontrollable factor" is within the organization's

control, in most cases, and should be addressed as a risk reduction strategy.

Concrete questions about each function mentioned above can help team members reach the essence of the problem—the systems that lie behind or underneath problematic processes. At this stage, questions can be worded in the form of "To what degree does ... ?" Follow-up questions for each could be "Can this be improved, and if so, how?" and "What are the pros and cons of expending the necessary resources to improve this?" See Sidebar 5-1, pages 90–91, for a full itemization of possible questions.

Other questions may emerge in the course of an analysis. All questions should be fully considered. One team investigating a patient suicide found that systems involving human resources, information management, environmental management, and leadership issues were found to be root causes of the sentinel event:
- In the human resources area, age-specific staff competence had not been assessed adequately and staff needed additional training in management of suicidal patients.
- In the information management area, information about the patient's past admission was not available. Communication delays resulted in failure to implement appropriate preventive actions.
- In the environmental management area, the team found that access to the appropriate unit for the patient was denied.

Checklist 5-1, pages 92–93, might provide a handy way to ensure that the team has considered selected system-based issues. Readers might wish to refer back to Figure 1-2, page 14, in Chapter 1 for a list of the systems or processes that should be considered and investigated for each type of sentinel event.

Another proposed classification system for causal factors is geared more to a manufacturing environment. However, it may be helpful to review this and other classification systems to ensure that the

Sidebar 5-1. Root Cause Analysis Questions

The following questions may be used to probe for systems problems that underlie problematic processes.

Questions concerning human resource issues may include the following:

- To what degree are staff members properly qualified and currently competent for their responsibilities? Can these be improved and, if so, how? What are the pros and cons of expending the necessary resources to improve these?

- How does actual staffing compare with ideal levels? Can this be improved and, if so, how? What are the pros and cons of expending the necessary resources to improve this?

- What are the plans for dealing with contingencies that would tend to reduce effective staffing levels? Can this be improved and, if so, how? What are the pros and cons of expending the necessary resources to improve this?

- To what degree is staff performance in the operant processes addressed? Can this be improved and, if so, how? What are the pros and cons of expending the necessary resources to improve this?

- How can orientation and in-service training be improved? What are the pros and cons of expending the necessary resources to improve this?

Questions concerning information management issues may include the following:

- To what degree is all necessary information

available when needed? What are the barriers to information availability and access? To what degree is the information accurate and complete? To what degree is the information unambiguous? Can these factors be improved and, if so, how? What are the pros and cons of expending the necessary resources to improve in this area?

- To what degree is the communication of information among participants adequate? Can this be improved and, if so, how? What are the pros and cons of expending the necessary resources to improve this?

Questions concerning environmental management issues may include the following:

- To what degree was the physical environment appropriate for the processes being carried out? Can this be improved and, if so, how? What are the pros and cons of expending the necessary resources to improve this?

- To what degree are systems in place to identify environmental risks? Can this be improved and, if so, how? What are the pros and cons of expending the necessary resources to improve this?

- What emergency and failure mode responses have been planned and tested? Can this be improved and, if so, how? What are the pros and cons of expending the necessary resources to improve this?

Questions concerning leadership issues may include the following:

- To what degree is the culture conducive to

Sidebar 5-1. Root Cause Analysis Questions (continued)

risk identification and reduction? Can this be improved and, if so, how? What are the pros and cons of expending the necessary resources to improve this?

- What are the barriers to communication of potential risk factors? Can this be improved and, if so, how? What are the pros and cons of expending the necessary resources to improve this?

- To what degree is the prevention of adverse outcomes communicated as a high priority? How is this communicated? Can this be improved and, if so, how? What are the pros and cons of expending the necessary resources to improve this?

Questions concerning uncontrollable factors may include the following:

- What can be done to protect against the effects of uncontrollable factors? What are the pros and cons of expending the necessary resources to improve this area?

---

team has identified all possible causal factors. This causal factor category list follows.[1]

Human Factors

- Verbal communication: the spoken presentation or exchange of information.
- Written procedures and documents: the written presentation or exchange of information.
- Man-machine interface: the design of equipment used to communicate information from the plan to a person.
- Environmental conditions: the physical conditions of a work area.
- Work schedule: factors that contribute to the ability

of the worker to perform his or her assigned task in an effective manner.

- Work practices: methods workers use to ensure safe and timely completion of a task.
- Work organization/planning: the work-related tasks, including planning, identifying the scope, assigning responsible individuals, and scheduling the task to be performed.
- Supervisory methods: techniques used to directly control work-related tasks; in particular, a method used to direct workers in the accomplishment of tasks.
- Training/qualification: how the training program was developed and the process of presenting information on how a task is to be performed prior to accomplishing the task.
- Change management: the process whereby the hardware or software associated with a particular operation, technique, or system is modified.
- Resource management: the process whereby manpower and material are allocated for a particular task/objective.
- Managerial methods: an administrative technique used to control or direct work-related plan activities, which includes the process whereby manpower and material are allocated for a particular objective.

Equipment Factors

- Design configuration and analysis: the design layout of systems or subsystems needed to support plan operation and maintenance.
- Equipment condition: the failure mechanism of the equipment is the physical cause of the failure.
- Environmental conditions: the physical conditions of the equipment area.
- Equipment specification, manufacture, and construction: the process that includes the manufacture and installation of equipment in the plant.
- Maintenance/testing: the process of maintaining components/systems in optimum conditions.
- Plant/system operation: the actual performance of the equipment or component when performing its intended function.

Checklist 5-1. Problematic Systems or Processes

Use this checklist to identify and rank problematic systems or processes. Use a "1" to indicate a problem that is a primary factor and a "2" to indicate a problem that could be considered a contributing factor.

Human Resources Issues

__ Qualifications of staff
  __ defined
  __ verified
  __ reviewed and updated on regular basis
__ Qualifications of physicians
  __ defined
  __ verified
  __ reviewed and updated on regular basis
__ Qualifications of agency staff
  __ defined
  __ verified
  __ reviewed and updated on regular basis
__ Training of staff
  __ adequacy of training program content
  __ receipt of necessary training
  __ competence/proficiency testing following training
__ Training of physicians
  __ adequacy of training program content
  __ receipt of necessary training
  __ competence/proficiency testing following training
__ Training of agency staff
  __ adequacy of training program content
  __ receipt of necessary training
  __ competence/proficiency testing following training
__ Competence of staff
  __ initially verified
  __ reviewed and verified on regular basis
__ Competence of physicians
  __ initially verified
  __ reviewed and verified on regular basis
__ Competence of agency staff
  __ initially verified
  __ reviewed and verified on regular basis
__ Supervision of staff
  __ adequate for new employees
  __ adequate for high-risk activities
__ Current staffing levels
  __ based on reasonable patient acuity measure
  __ based on reasonable workloads
__ Current scheduling practices
  __ overtime expectations
  __ time for work activities
  __ time between shifts for shift changes

Information Management Issues

__ Availability of information
__ Accuracy of information
__ Thoroughness of information
__ Clarity of information
__ Communication of information between relevant individuals/participants

Environmental Management Issues

__ Physical environment
  __ appropriateness to processes being carried out
  __ lighting
  __ temperature control
  __ noise control

Checklist 5-1. Problematic Systems or Processes (continued)

__ size/design of space
__ exposure to infection risks
__ cleanliness
__ Systems to identify environmental risks
__ Quality control activities
__ adequacy of procedures and techniques
__ inspections
__ Planned, tested, and implemented emergency and failure mode responses

Leadership and Communication Issues
__ Culture conducive to risk reduction
__ Corrective actions identified and implemented
__ Risk reduction initiatives receive priority attention
__ Barriers to communication of risks and errors
__ Communication
   __ present, as appropriate
   __ appropriate method
   __ understood
   __ timely
   __ adequate
__ Managerial controls and policies
   __ appropriate controls and policies in place
   __ policies enforced
   __ communication regarding policy changes

External Factor

- External: human or nonhuman influence outside the usual control of the company.

10 Step Ten: Prune the List of Root Causes

The team's list of causal factors may be lengthy. Regardless of its length or the technique used, the team should analyze each cause or factor. This involves using reasoning skills based on logic. Asking two questions will help to clarify whether each cause or problem listed is actually a true root cause:

- "If we fix this problem, will the problem recur in the future?" and
- "If this problem is a root cause, how does it explain what happened or what could have happened?"

One method is using three criteria to determine if each cause is a root cause or a secondary or contributing cause:[2]

- The problem would not have occurred had the cause not been present;
- The problem will not recur due to the same causal factor if the cause is corrected or eliminated; and
- Correction or elimination of the cause will prevent recurrence of similar conditions.

If these statements are converted to positive questions and a "no" answer is obtained, the problem is a root cause. If a "yes" answer is obtained, the problem is a contributing cause. Again, it may be helpful to develop a checklist with these questions built in.

A sample checklist with the questions appears as Checklist 5-2, page 94.

11 Step Eleven: Confirm Root Causes and Consider Their Interrelationships

It is highly likely that the team will identify more than one root cause for the sentinel event or near miss. Even in those very rare instances when a sentinel event results from an intentional act of an individual, more than one root cause is likely (for example,

Checklist 5-2. Differentiating Root Causes and Contributing Causes

To differentiate root causes from contributing causes, ask the following questions of each of the causes on the team's list. If the answer is no to each of the three questions, the cause is a root cause. If the answer is yes to any one of the three questions, the cause is a contributing cause.

Cause #1 _____

Would the problem have occurred if Cause #1 had not been present?
☐ No = root cause   ☐ Yes = contributing cause

Will the problem recur due to the same causal factor if Cause #1 is corrected or eliminated?
☐ No = root cause   ☐ Yes = contributing cause

Will correction or elimination of Cause #1 lead to similar events?
☐ No = root cause   ☐ Yes = contributing cause

Cause #2 _____

Would the problem have occurred if Cause #2 had not been present?
☐ No = root cause   ☐ Yes = contributing cause

Will the problem recur due to the same causal factor if Cause #2 is corrected or eliminated?
☐ No = root cause   ☐ Yes = contributing cause

Will correction or elimination of Cause #2 lead to similar events?
☐ No = root cause   ☐ Yes = contributing cause

Cause #3 _____

Would the problem have occurred if Cause #3 had not been present?
☐ No = root cause   ☐ Yes = contributing cause

Will the problem recur due to the same causal factor if Cause #3 is corrected or eliminated?
☐ No = root cause   ☐ Yes = contributing cause

Will correction or elimination of Cause #3 lead to similar events?
☐ No = root cause   ☐ Yes = contributing cause

personnel screening, communication, and so forth). Sentinel events in industry tend to have two to four root causes and these root causes tend to be interrelated. To date, the Joint Commission's Sentinel Event Database indicates four to six root causes identified by participating organizations for each sentinel event.

For example, organizations that experienced a sentinel event related to **restraint use** reviewed by the Joint Commission identified the following root causes:[3]

- Staffing issues, including insufficient staff orientation, training, competence assessment, or credentialing or insufficient staffing levels;
- Unsafe equipment or equipment use, such as use of split side rails without side rail protectors, use of a high-neck vest, incorrect application of a restraining device, or a monitor or an alarm not working or not being used when appropriate;
- Lack of adequate observation procedures or practices;
- Inadequate assessment, including incomplete examination of the individual to identify contraband, such as matches, that could result in fire and harm to the individual; and
- Inadequate care planning, such as alternatives to restraints not fully considered, restraints used as punishment, and inappropriate room or unit assignment.

More than 90% of the organizations cited insufficient staff orientation and training as a root cause, 80% cited equipment-related factors, and 65% cited lack of observation procedures or practices for individuals served.

Organizations that experienced **suicides** in a 24-hour care setting reviewed by the Joint Commission identified the following root causes:[4]

- The environment of care, such as the presence of nonbreakaway bars, rods, or safety rails; lack of testing of breakaway hardware; and inadequate security;

- Patient assessment methods, such as incomplete suicide risk assessment at intake, absent or incomplete reassessment, and incomplete examination of the individual (for example, failure to identify contraband);
- Staff-related factors, such as insufficient orientation or training, incomplete competency review or credentialing, and inadequate staffing levels;
- Incomplete or infrequent patient observations;
- Information-related factors, such as incomplete communication among caregivers and information being unavailable when needed; and
- Care planning, such as assignment of the patient to an inappropriate unit or location.

Organizations that experienced **infant abductions or release to wrong families** reviewed by the Joint Commission identified the following root causes:[5]

- Security equipment factors, such as security equipment not being available, operational, or used as intended;
- Physical environmental factors, such as no line of sight to entry points as well as unmonitored elevator or stairwell access to postpartum and nursery areas;
- Inadequate patient education;
- Staff-related factors, such as insufficient orientation/training, competency/credentialing issues, and insufficient staffing levels;
- Information management-related factors, such as birth information published in local newspapers, delay in notifying security when an abduction was suspected, improper communication of relevant information among caregivers, and improper communication between hospital units; and
- Organizational culture factors such as reluctance to confront unidentified visitors/providers.

Root causes of **medication errors** include orientation/training, communication, storage/access issues, information availability, competency/credentialing, supervision, labeling, and distraction.

Root causes of **wrong-site surgery** include miscommunication by the operating room team, incomplete patient assessment, failure to follow or the lack of a verification policy, operating room hierarchy, failure to communicate with the patient, lack of available information, distraction, and competency/credentialing issues.

Root causes of death or serious injury due to **treatment delays** include inadequate communication among caregivers, insufficient staff orientation and training or insufficient staffing, inadequate assessment, inadequate information management, and faulty equipment.

Root causes of sentinel events related to **patient falls** include inadequate caregiver communication; inadequate assessment and reassessment; inadequate care planning and provision; inadequate staffing, orientation, training, and supervision; and an unsafe environment of care.

Although this information may provide insight into areas to explore, organizations should not rely exclusively on these lists, but should uncover their own unique root causes.

The identification of *all* root causes is essential to preventing a failure or near miss. Why? Because the interaction of the root causes is likely to be "at the root" of the problem. If an organization eliminates one root cause only, it has reduced the likelihood of that one very specific adverse outcome occurring again. But if the organization misses the other five root causes, it is possible that those root causes could interact in another way to cause a different but equally adverse outcome. The root causes collectively represent, in effect, latent conditions that could occur. *Latent conditions* are, in effect, accidents or sentinel events waiting to happen. The combination of root causes sets the stage for sentinel events. Effective identification of *all* of the root causes and an understanding of their interaction can aid organizations in changing processes to eliminate a whole family of risks, not just a single risk. Elimination of only one of the root causes

mentioned above will not eliminate the risk inherent in the processes addressing restraint use, the prevention of suicide in a 24-hour care setting, infant abduction, or other sentinel events.

For example, with the restraint use case, to eliminate the root cause "unsafe equipment use," staff can be trained in selecting safe equipment and using it safely. However, what happens six months later when an individual staff member has forgotten how to use a four-point restraint properly? Does the organization have an effective plan for assessing the continued competence of the staff member to use restraint safely and to provide follow-up training when necessary? What happens if restraint is required when agency staff are on duty? Are they trained and competent to use restraint safely? After an individual is placed in restraint, does the staff member know how to consistently observe the individual in restraint according to organization policies and procedures (for example, to *detect* the result of a mistake in the restraint application process or an equipment failure)? Each of the root causes is interrelated to others. Elimination of a single root cause will not eliminate the latent conditions waiting to happen.

If the team identifies more than six root causes, a number of the causes may be defined too specifically. In this case, the team may wish to review whether one or more of the root causes could logically be combined with another to reflect more basic, system-oriented causes. The team should verify each of the remaining root causes. This involves cross-checking for accuracy and consistency all facts and all tools and techniques used to analyze information. Any inconsistencies and discrepancies should be resolved.

How does the organization know whether and when it has identified *all* of the true root causes of a sentinel event? Try using a checklist for determining whether the team has identified all the root causes. The team will want to report its root cause findings to the leaders of its organization. Leaders must be informed, as should the individuals likely to be impacted by changes emerging from the findings during the next stage of the root cause analysis. See Chapter 6, pages 124–126, for more information on communicating the results of the team's efforts.

References

1.   Ammerman M: *The Root Cause Analysis Handbook: A Simplified Approach to Identifying, Correcting, and Reporting Workplace Errors. New York*: Quality Resources, 1998, pp 66–67.

2.   Ammerman, pp 68–69.

3.   Joint Commission: Preventing restraint deaths. *Sentinel Event Alert*, Issue 8, Nov 18, 1998.

4.   Joint Commission: Inpatient suicides: Recommendations for prevention. *Sentinel Event Alert*, Issue 7, Nov 6, 1998.

5.   Joint Commission: Infant abductions: Preventing future occurrences. *Sentinel Event Alert*, Issue 9, Apr 9, 1999.

Worksheet 5-1. Probing for Underlying Causes

The team might find it helpful to use a worksheet that helps it probe for the underlying causes of proximate causes. For example, with the fire-related death of a restrained patient, the worksheet could be organized (and begun) as follows:

Proximate Causes   **Underlying Causes**

1. Missed observation   Staff training and orientation

                                                   Staffing model

2. Patient possessed contraband matches   Patient observation procedures

                                                   Suicide risk assessment procedure

3. _____   _____

   _____   _____

   _____   _____

   _____   _____

4. _____   _____

   _____   _____

   _____   _____

   _____   _____

5. _____   _____

   _____   _____

   _____   _____

Chapter 6

Designing and Implementing an Action Plan for Improvement

In previous chapters, identifying the proximate and root causes of a sentinel event or near miss event was discussed. The final and perhaps most important stage of the root cause analysis process involves identifying risk reduction strategies, setting priorities and objectives for improvement in areas identified as "at the root of the problem," and developing, implementing, and measuring the effectiveness of improvement efforts. This chapter covers these topics in workbook format. Again, Figure 1-3, pages 18–20, from Chapter 1 provides the framework for this step of the analysis.

Step 1: Organize a Team
Step 2: Define the Problem
Step 3: Study the Problem
Step 4: Determine What Happened
Step 5: Identify Contributing Process Factors
Step 6: Identify Other Contributing Factors
Step 7: Measure—Collect and Assess Data on Proximate and Underlying Causes
Step 8: Design and Implement Interim Changes
Step 9: Identify Which Systems Are Involved— The Root Causes
Step 10: Prune the List of Root Causes
Step 11: Confirm Root Causes and Consider Their Interrelationships
Step 12: Explore and Identify Risk Reduction Strategies
Step 13: Formulate Improvement Actions
Step 14: Evaluate Proposed Improvement Actions
Step 15: Design Improvements
Step 16: Ensure Acceptability of the Action Plan
Step 17: Implement the Improvement Plan
Step 18: Develop Measures of Effectiveness and Ensure Their Success
Step 19: Evaluate Implementation of Improvement Efforts
Step 20: Take Additional Action
Step 21: Communicate the Results

12 Step Twelve: Explore and Identify Risk Reduction Strategies

The team asks, "So what are we going to do with the problematic systems now that we have identified them?" Once the team has a solid hypothesis about one or more root causes, the next step is to explore and identify risk reduction strategies to help ensure that faulty systems are improved for the future.

The team might start by exploring relevant literature on risk reduction and error-prevention strategies. Much has been written about the engineering approach to failure prevention and how it differs from the medical approach. Some of the literature's key points are described here.

The pervasive view of errors in the engineering field is that humans err frequently and that the cause of an error is often beyond the individual's control. In designing systems and processes, engineers begin with the premise that anything can and will go wrong. Their role is a proactive one—to design accordingly. Because engineering-based industries do not expect individuals to perform flawlessly, they try to design systems that make it difficult for individuals to make mistakes. By compensating for less-than-perfect human performance, engineering systems achieve a high degree of reliability through backup systems and designed redundancy. A failure rate even as low as 1% is not tolerated. The emphasis is on systems rather than individuals.

In contrast, the still-pervasive view in the health care field is that errors are the result of individual human failure and that humans generally perform flawlessly. Hence, processes in health care organizations tend to be designed based on the premise that nothing will go wrong. Education and training, more extensive in health care than in most other fields, focus on teaching professionals to do the right thing. The assumption is that properly educated and trained health care professionals will not make mistakes. Those that do are retrained, punished, or sanctioned. The immediate causes of errors are identified and corrected, but not planned or designed for. Root causes are rarely identified.

Lucian L. Leape, MD, has done much work comparing risk reduction approaches in various industries to those in the health care industry. He suggests four safety design characteristics from the aviation industry that could, with some modification, prove useful in improving safety in the health care industry:[1]

- Built-in multiple buffers, automation, and redundancy. Instrumentation in airplane cockpits includes multiple and purposely redundant monitoring instruments. The design systems assume that errors and failures are inevitable and should be absorbed.
- Standardized procedures. Protocols that must be followed exist for operating and maintaining airplanes.

- A highly developed and rigidly enforced training, examination, and certification process. Pilots take proficiency exams every six months.
- Institutionalized safety. The airline industry reports directly to two agencies that regulate all aspects of flying, prescribe safety procedures, and investigate all accidents. A confidential safety reporting system established by the Federal Aviation Administration enables pilots, controllers, or others to report dangerous situations, including errors they have made, to a third party without penalty. This program greatly increases error reporting in aviation, resulting in enhanced communication and prompt problem solving.

An error-prevention strategy for the health care industry must include designing systems to absorb failures, standardizing tasks and processes to minimize reliance on weak aspects of cognition, testing of professional performance, and institutionalizing safety through "near miss" and nonpunitive reporting. For example, clinical practice guidelines and organization policies and protocols, designed to reduce variation in the care provided by practitioners, can help to reduce the likelihood of failures.

Risk reduction strategies must emphasize a systems rather than an individual human approach. A system can be thought of as any collection of components and the relationships among them, whether the components are human or not, when the components have been brought together for a well-defined goal or purpose.[2] As Leape writes, "Creating a safe process, whether it be flying an airplane, running a hospital, or performing cardiac surgery, requires attention to methods of error reduction at each stage of system development: design, construction, maintenance, allocation of resources, training, and development of operational procedures."[3] If errors are made, if deficiencies are discovered, individuals at each stage must revisit previous decisions and redesign or reorganize the process.

Designing for safety means making it difficult for humans to err. However, those designing systems must recognize that failures will occur and that recovery or correction should be built into the system. If this is not possible, failures must be able to be detected promptly so that individuals have time to take corrective actions. For example, preoperative labeling of surgical sites, a check by the circulating nurse, and checks conducted directly with the patient and family facilitate the detection of potential wrong-site surgical errors.

Risk points—specific points in a process that are susceptible to failure or system breakdown—must be eliminated through design or redesign efforts (see Chapter 3, page 52). Built-in buffers and redundancy, task and process simplification and standardization, and training are all appropriate design mechanisms to reduce the likelihood of failure at risk points and elsewhere.

For example, prior to the administration of medications, multiple and redundant checks, such as asking the patient his or her name, checking the patient's armband, and so forth can help confirm that the drug will be given to the right patient. See Sidebar 6-1, page 102, for risk points for medication errors and risk reduction strategies to prevent such failures.

Risk points and/or risk reduction strategies for wrong-site surgery, restraint-related deaths, suicide, and infant abductions or release to wrong families follow. Readers should note that a number of these strategies are not specific Joint Commission requirements, but are presented for consideration by all health care organizations.

Risk points for **wrong-site surgery** include the following:
- Communication before reaching operating suite;
- Communication in operating suite;
- Hierarchical issues of communication;
- Communication with patient/family;
- Information availability;
- Multiple surgery sites;
- Conflicting chart information;

- Confused patient; and
- X ray quality/accuracy.

Risk reduction strategies to reduce the likelihood of failures associated with *preoperative procedures* include the following:
- Mark operative site;
- Require surgeon to obtain informed consent;
- Require preoperative verification by surgeon, anesthesiologist/anesthetist, and patient or family;
- Personally review X rays; and
- Revise equipment setup procedures.

To reduce the likelihood of failures in the *operating suite*:
- Verify before prep and drape;
- Prep signature inside field;
- Time-out verbal verification; and
- Confirm by "bone bite" or fluoroscopy.

Risk points for **restraint use** include the following:
- Restraining patients with high risk factors, including those who smoke, those with deformities that preclude proper fit of restraint, and those with potentially compromised protective reflexes (such as those under conscious sedation or those profoundly intoxicated);
- Restraining patients in supine position (may increase risk of aspiration);
- Restraining patients in prone position (may increase risk of suffocation); and
- Restraining patients in room not under continuous observation.

Risk reduction strategies include the following:
- Do not restrain patient in bed with unprotected, split side rails;
- Use appropriate restraint for person, age, and goal;
- Never use a towel, bag, or cover over an individual's face;
- Ensure that all smoking materials are removed from individual's access;
- Continuously observe any individual who is restrained;

Sidebar 6-1. Medication Errors: Risk Points and Risk Reduction Strategies

Risk Points or Common Causes
- Inadequate training/education
- Competence (lapses in performance, failure to comply with policies and procedures)
- Supervision
- Staffing (excessive workload, incorrect mix)
- Communication failures
- Distraction due to environmental issues
- Information availability
- Medication storage/access
- Labeling
- Nomenclature
- Dosage calculation
- Equipment failure
- Abbreviations
- Handwriting

Risk Reduction Strategies
To reduce the likelihood of failures associated with *prescribing* errors:
- Implement a system of computerized order entry by physicians (to decrease the likelihood of dosage error, prompt for allergies, and provide information on drug-drug and drug-food interactions); and
- Redefine the role of pharmacists to enable them to perform daily rounds with physicians, work with registered nurses, and serve as on-site resources.

To reduce the likelihood of failures associated with *dispensing*:
- Do not rely on color-coding;
- Remove look-alikes;
- Use bar codes if possible;
- Avoid lethal medications in bolus form;
- Use premixed solutions, when possible;
- Minimize supplier/product changes;

- Use auxiliary labels (such as, "for IM [intramuscular] only");
- Support questioning of unclear orders; and
- Eliminate guessing.

To reduce the likelihood of failures associated with *access* to medications:
- Remove high-risk medications from care units;
- Label high-risk medications as such; and
- Establish and implement policies and procedures for use of off-hours pharmacy.

To reduce the likelihood of failures associated with *medication delivery*:
- Be sure that equipment defaults to least harmful mode;
- Use automated pharmacy units as a tool for improving the process, not an inherent solution; and
- Recognize that polypharmacy equals higher risk.

To reduce the likelihood of failures associated with *human resources and competence factors*:
- Address education and training issues (orientation, competence assessment, and training with new medications and devices);
- Support professional ethics and judgment;
- Implement systems involving double checks;
- Make safe staffing choices;
- Tackle illegible handwriting;
- Discourage use of acronyms and abbreviations;
- Control availability of high-risk drugs;
- Address environmental issues (tackle distraction and its impact);
- Standardize medication times; and
- Use patients as safety partners.

- Educate staff on appropriate use and alternative measures;
- Revise staffing model;
- Ensure staff competence and training;
- Use less restrictive measures, increase and standardize choices; and
- Revise policy and procedure regarding assessment.

Strategies to reduce the risk of **suicide** in a 24-hour care setting include the following:
- Revise assessment/reassessment procedures and assure adherence;
- Update staffing model;
- Educate staff on suicide risk factors;
- Update policies on patient observation;
- Monitor consistency of implementation;
- Revise information transfer procedures;
- Revisit contraband polices;
- Identify and remove nonbreakaway hardware;
- Weight-test all breakaway hardware;
- Redesign or retrofit security measures;
- Educate family and friends on suicide risk factors;
- Consider patients in all areas;
- Ensure that staff members ask about suicidal thoughts every shift;
- Be cautious at times of change (admission, discharge, passes);
- Avoid reliance on pacts;
- Be suspicious if symptoms lighten suddenly; and
- Involve all staff in the solutions.

Strategies to reduce the risk of **infant abductions or release to wrong families** include the following:
- Develop and implement a proactive infant abduction prevention plan;
- Include information on visitor/provider identification as well as identification of potential abductors/abduction situations during staff orientation and in-service curriculum programs;
- Enhance parent education concerning abduction risks and parent responsibility for reducing risk and then assess the parents' level of understanding;
- Attach secure identically numbered bands to the

baby (wrist and ankle bands), mother, and father or significant other immediately after birth;
- Footprint the baby, take a color photograph of the baby, and record the baby's physical examination within two hours of birth;
- Require staff to wear up-to-date, conspicuous, color photograph identification badges;
- Discontinue publication of birth notices in local newspapers;
- Consider options for controlling access to nursery/postpartum unit such as swipe-card locks, keypad locks, entry point alarms or video surveillance (any locking systems must comply with fire codes); and
- Consider implementing an infant security tag or abduction alarm system.

Systems engineering literature includes numerous other design concepts that could be useful tools to prevent failures and sentinel events in health care organizations. *Redundancy* is one such concept familiar to the aerospace and nuclear power industries, where systems have backups and even the backups normally have backups. System reliability can be increased by introducing redundancy into system design. However, the cost of designing in redundancy is an issue in most health care environments. The engineering literature also describes the benefits of simplification, standardization, and loose coupling to reduce the possibility of systems-related problems.

Fail-safe design is also a concept familiar to high-reliability industries, including aerospace and nuclear engineering. The design may be fail-passive, fail-operational, or fail-active. For example, a circuit breaker is a fail-passive device that opens when a dangerous situation occurs, thereby making an electrical system safe. A destruct system on a satellite or an air-to-air missile is an example of a fail-active device. If the satellite or missile misses its target within a set time, the destruct system blows the satellite or missile apart to halt its flight and limit any damage it might cause by falling to the ground.

Checklist 6-1, right, provides the key risk reduction strategies suggested in the medical and engineering literature.

Failure mode and effects analysis (FMEA) can also be used to identify risk reduction opportunities. Also known in the literature as failure mode, effects, and criticality analysis (FMECA), FMEA offers a systematic way of examining a design prospectively for possible ways in which failure can occur. Potential failures are identified in terms of failure "modes" or symptoms, as opposed to causes. For each failure mode, the effects on the total system or process are studied. Actions (planned or already taken) can be reviewed for their potential to minimize the probability of failure or the effects of failure. FMEA's goal is to prevent poor results, which in health care means "harm to patients." Its greatest strength lies in its ability to focus users on the process of redesigning potentially problematic processes to prevent the occurrence of failures.

Although the technique has been used very effectively in the engineering world since the 1960s, its use in the health care world began as late as the 1990s. FMEA is now gaining broader acceptance in health care as a tool for prospective analysis due to the efforts of the Joint Commission, the Department of Veterans Affairs' National Center for Patient Safety (NCPS), and the Institute for Safe Medication Practices (ISMP), among others. In 2002 the Joint Commission published the first book on FMEA's application in health care[4] which is intended as a companion publication to this publication. The eight steps involved in an FMEA approach, as outlined by the Joint Commission, appear in Chapter 7, page 153.

One impetus for FMEA's broader acceptance is the Joint Commission's patient safety and medical/health care error reduction requirements, which require leaders to define and implement a proactive system for identifying risk and reducing medical and health care errors. The requirement outlines the use of FMEA. Proactive risk reduction processes that encompass the basic steps included in an FMEA approach may be used to comply

---

Checklist 6-1. Identifying Risk Reduction Strategies

To reduce the likelihood of failures, the medical and engineering literature offers the following tips:
- ☐ Use an engineering approach to failure prevention.
- ☐ Start with the premise that anything can and will go wrong.
- ☐ Design systems that make the safest thing to do the easiest thing to do.
- ☐ Design systems that make it difficult for individuals to err.
- ☐ Build in as much redundancy as possible.
- ☐ Use fail-safe design whenever possible.
- ☐ Simplify and standardize procedures.
- ☐ Automate procedures.
- ☐ Ensure rigidly enforced training and competence assessment processes.
- ☐ Ensure nonpunitive reporting of near misses.
- ☐ Eliminate risk points.

---

with Joint Commission requirements. The requirement was effective for hospitals July 1, 2001, and will be effective for other types of health care organizations accredited by the Joint Commission in forthcoming years.

FMEA is described here because root cause analysis teams may also wish to use FMEA to proactively identify risk reduction opportunities during their root cause analysis of a sentinel event or near miss.

Tool: *Failure mode and effects analysis (FMEA)*

A performance improvement team at a community hospital in Michigan used failure mode and effects analysis for one of the first times in health care to proactively analyze and reduce medication errors associated with potassium chloride (KCl).[5] The focus was on developing strategies to reduce the risk of future fatal errors. The team followed the steps outlined in Table 6-1, right.

The process flow diagram developed by the team for the medication use process from point of initiation through completion appears as Figure 6-1, page 106. The team's outline of what could go wrong and its ranking appears as Table 6-2, page 107. Possible error-preventing actions appear in Table 6-3, page 108. These are presented as a model to help teams successfully integrate a ranking system.

13 Step Thirteen: Formulate Improvement Actions

With the list of root causes in hand, the team is now ready to start devising potential solutions to systems-related problems. Known as corrective or improvement actions, these solutions are required to prevent a problem from occurring or recurring due to the same root cause(s) or interaction of root causes. The team may include the same members as during the early stages of the root cause analysis, or new members might be brought on board as required by the recommended improvements.

When formulating improvement actions, think in terms of the everyday work of the organization. Work can be defined in terms of functions or processes. A function is a group of processes with a common goal, and a process is a series of linked, goal-directed activities. Improvement actions should be directed primarily at processes. As stated earlier in this book, process improvement holds the greatest opportunity for signifi-cant change, whereas changes related to an individ-ual's performance tend to have limited effect. Good people often find themselves carrying out bad process-es. System problems identified and resolutions suggest-ed by an interdisciplinary medication incident task force at one organization appear as Table 6-4, page 109. Returning to the sentinel events described in Chapter

Table 6-1.
Steps in Failure Mode and Effects Analysis

1. Set up a process flow diagram.
2. Retrace the process flow diagram, assuming the worst, to figure out what could go wrong along the way.
3. Decide what the effects of failure might be on the remainder of the process.
4. Rank the estimated possibility of occurrence using the following scale: 1=remote possibility; 5=possibility; and 10=almost certain.
5. Rank the estimated severity of the overall failure using the following scale: 1=will not cause patient harm; 5=may affect patient adversely; and 10=injury or death will occur.
6. Rank the estimated likelihood that failure will be detected before accident takes place: 1=will always be detected; 5=might be detected; and 10=detection not possible.
7. Calculate the "criticality index" (mean of steps 4, 5, and 6).
8. Decide on interventions to lower the criticality index.
9. Take action.
10. Assess.

Source: Cohen M: Failure mode and effects analysis: Dealing with human error in medicine. *Proceedings of the Physicians Insurance Company of Michigan.* Apr 1994.

3 on pages 46–47, consider the following examples of how root cause analysis teams could approach the identification of improvement actions.

In the **suicide** example, the team has completed a cause-and-effect diagram indicating multiple system problems, including assessment of suicide risk, environment of care, and emergency procedures. The

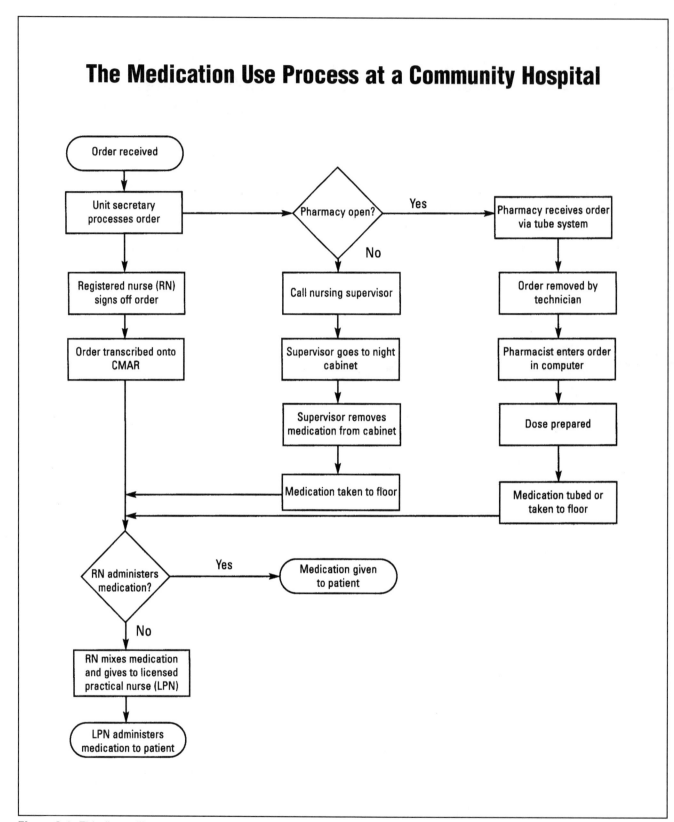

Figure 6-1. This figure illustrates the simplified process flowchart one community hospital created as step 1 in a failure mode and effects analysis. In step 2 they went through the flowchart, action by action, to brainstorm what might go wrong. Table 6-2 on page 107 lists the possible failures the hospital brainstormed. CMAR, computerized medication administration record.

Source: Fletcher CE: Failure and effects analysis. *J Nurs Adm* 27(12):23, 1997.

Table 6-2. Possible Risk Points in the Medication Use Process

Order Received
- Phone order not clarified.
- Verbal order not clarified.
- Written order illegible.
- Dose may be incorrect.
- Incorrect route.
- Order written on wrong chart.
- Order written on right chart, but stamped with wrong name.
- Wrong drug.
- Drug not indicated.
- Language barrier present with verbal phone order.

Unit Secretary Processes Order
- Does not take order out of chart.
- Sends order to department other than pharmacy.
- Misplaces order and does not send it at all.
- Misinterprets and thus processes incorrectly.
- Delays in processing occur.
- Stamps wrong name on order sheet.

Registered Nurse Signs Off Order
- Delays order.
- Does not read order carefully, but processes it anyway.
- Does not take time to read order, but processes it anyway.
- Cosigns order without giving it to secretary; does not go through correct process.
- Cannot read/misreads order.
- Orders added by physician after initial order processed; RN does not see additional orders.
- Unfamiliar with drug: allergy, dose, and/or cross sensitivity.

Order Transcribed onto CMAR
- RN's handwriting unclear.
- Order transcribed onto wrong computerized medical administration record (CMAR).
- Order transcribed incorrectly.
- Order not transcribed in a timely manner.
- Lack of nursing communication to RN or licensed practical nurse (LPN) giving medication.
- Forgetting/failure to transcribe.

RN Mixes Medication
- Miscalculated dose.
- Miscalculated measurement of volume.
- Selects wrong drug.
- Prepares wrong drug brought by supervisor (after hours).
- Does not match the order to the chart.
- Labeling errors: drug is not actually added to IV or IV contains drug but no label.
- Lacks knowledge of administration policies and procedures.
- Lacks knowledge regarding IV versus oral dosing guidelines.
- Interrupted during preparation.
- Lacks routine/organization when doing the task.

RN or LPN Administers Medication to Patient
- Wrong patient.
- Incorrect labeling.
- Intravenous accurate control (IVAC) not used.
- No IVAC available.
- Wrong rate of flow set on IVAC.

Source: Fletcher CE: Failure and effects analysis. *J Nurs Adm* 27(12):24, 1997.

Table 6-3. Possible Failure-Preventing Actions

Remove Alternatives
- Eliminate dangerous items and procedures.
- Limit use or access.
- Locate items with care.
- Follow protocols and procedures.
- Ascertain certification or privileging.
- Maintain hospital drug formulary control.
- Avoid potential for "confirmation bias" (minimize look-alike containers, names, computer abbreviations, and so forth).
- Minimize consequence of error.

Improve Detection
- Orientation, education, and additional training.
- Protocols and procedures.
- Redundancy.
- "Lock and key" design.

- Hazard warnings and signs, auxiliary labels, medication administration record (MAR) warnings, and so forth.
- Technology (bar code, computer, and so forth).
- Improved detection process.
- Documentation.
- Tactile cues.

Prevent Completion of Actions
- Fail-safe design.
- "Lock and key" design.
- Technology.

Minimize Consequence of Failure
- Reduce supply (volume, concentration, number of tablets, vials, and so forth).
- Modify defaults.

Source: Cohen M: Failure mode and effects analysis: Dealing with human error in medicine. *Proceedings of the Physicians Insurance Company of Michigan.* Apr 1994.

team might break into smaller subgroups. One group, including the psychiatrist, medical staff leader, and nurse, would address the failed patient assessment process. They might start by reviewing the current standard for assessment of suicide risk and how this standard is communicated in the behavioral health unit. Another group, including the administrator and plant safety representative, might start working on environment of care issues such as nonbreakaway showerheads. Another group, including emergency department physicians and the nursing staff, might work on emergency procedures.

In the **elopement** example, the root cause analysis team has identified multiple system problems including an unsafe environment of care, inadequate assessment and reassessment, and inadequate staff orientation, training and ongoing competence assessment. One subgroup, including the safety director, a nurse from the unit, and a social worker, might address possible actions to improve the long term care organization's security and safety measures. Another small group, including the medical director, director of nursing, activity staff member, and unit staff nurse, might address opportunities to improve the process used to assess and reassess individuals at risk for elopement. Another group, including the medical director, the director of nursing, and the performance improvement coordinator, might address strategies to ensure that staff know elopement risk factors and who is at risk for elopement and are assessed regularly for competence in identifying and caring for at-risk individuals.

Table 6-4. Sample System Problems and Suggested Resolutions

Problem

- Lack of uniform procedures in medication administration from one unit to another.
- Limited pharmacy involvement in the medication incident reporting and tracking process.
- Controlled drugs frequently involved in ordered drug errors.
- Use of unofficial abbreviations for drug names identified as a source of several unordered drug errors.
- Use of Latin abbreviations such as QD, QOD, and OD and abbreviation U for units identified as a source of errors.
- Physician order sheets were not removed from patients' charts, therefore pharmacy Kardex was not complete and accurate.

Suggested Resolution

- Assess current unit differences in medication administration procedures by developing a survey instrument. Determine methods to standardize procedures to minimize errors.
- Analyze weekly summary of errors, prepared in the Department of Pharmacy, to determine system defects that may be correctable.
- Investigate automated dispensing systems to minimize errors with controlled substances.
- Form a subcommittee of the Pharmacy and Therapeutics Committee to review this issue and recommend appropriate action.
- Organize subcommittee of the Pharmacy and Therapeutics Committee to prepare recommendation on use of abbreviations.
- Collect data to identify areas where this is most common; provide corrective measures to focus on these areas.

Source: Bradbury K, et al: Prevention of medication errors: Developing a continuous-quality improvement approach. *Mt Sinai J Med* 60(5):382, 1993.

In the **treatment delay** example, the team has identified system problems that led to the missed diagnosis of metastasized breast cancer. These include communication problems between caregivers, insufficient staff orientation and training, and inadequate information management. Subgroups of the ambulatory care organization's team probe each of these areas for improvement opportunities, looking at such issues as care documentation and the availability of clinical records, the timeliness and thoroughness of initial and regular reassessments, and shift-to-shift communication of information related to patient needs.

In the **medication error** example, the root cause analysis team has identified communication of medication orders and the failure to ensure safe medication storage and access as two key problems, among others. A subgroup, including the information technology staff member, the pharmacist, medical director, and a home health nurse, might investigate possible strategies to improve the accuracy of orders communicated to local pharmacies. Another subgroup, including the nursing supervisor, pharmacy supplier, home health nurse, and medical director, might investigate strategies to guard against medication theft and ensure proper implementation of the home health agency's medication administration policies and procedures.

For each root cause, the team should work together interactively either as a whole or in smaller groups to develop a list of possible improvement actions. Brainstorming can be used to generate additional ideas. The emphasis at this point is on generating as many improvement actions as possible, not on evaluating the ideas or their feasibility. The number of suggested improvement actions may vary based on the nature of the root cause and how it relates to other root causes. To ensure as thorough a list as possible, the team may wish to review the analyses of information used to identify root causes. Remember to encourage any and all ideas without critiquing them. In the hands of a skilled facilitator, even the seemingly wildest idea can lead to an effective improvement action during later stages of the analysis. Tools used, such as flowcharts or cause-and-effect diagrams, can prompt additional solutions. Ask questions of the group, such as the following:

- What might fix this problem?
- What other solutions can we generate?
- What other ideas haven't we thought of?

Tools: *Brainstorming, flowchart, cause-and-effect diagram*

Wilson and his colleagues suggest using the scientific method to develop a list of potential solutions. He restates the scientific method in terms of steps used in developing solutions:

- Become familiar with all the aspects of the problem and its causes;
- Derive a number of tentative solutions;
- Assemble as much detail as is needed to clearly define what it will require to implement these solutions;
- Evaluate the suggested solutions;
- Objectively test and revise the solutions; and
- Develop a final list of potential solutions.[6]

These steps may assist the team through the process of both developing and evaluating improvement actions.

14 Step Fourteen: Evaluate Proposed Improvement Actions

When the list of possible improvement actions is as complete as possible, the team is ready to evaluate the alternatives and select those actions to be recommended to leadership.

To begin the evaluation process, the team will want to rank the ideas based on criteria defined by the team. Gathering appropriate data is critical to this process. A simple six-point scale ranging from a low rank of 0 for "worst alternative" to a high rank of 5 for "best alternative" can be used at this point. To rank the proposed solutions, Ammerman suggests using criteria such as compatibility with other organization commitments and possible creation of other adverse effects.[7]

Initially, to prevent "group think," it is a good idea to ask each team member to rank the ideas on his or her own. The rankings can then be consolidated into a team ranking. To keep track of suggested improvement actions, complete Worksheet 6-1, page 127. Record the rankings assigned by individual team members and the team as a whole.

Failure mode and effects analysis may be a helpful tool at this point in the process. FMEA involves evaluating potential problems (or improvement actions) and prioritizing or ranking these on a proactive basis according to criteria defined by a team (see Table 6-1, page 105, and Chapter 7, page 153).

Tool: *Failure mode and effects analysis*

At the very least, every improvement action proposed by the team should be objective and measurable. If it is objective, implementation will be easier and those affected by the change are more likely to be receptive. If it is measurable, the team can ensure that improvement actually occurs. See Sidebar 6-2, page 111, for evaluative criteria for improvement actions. Before ranking the actions, ensure that the team reaches a consensus on which criteria are most relevant to the organization. Ranking the proposed ideas according to multiple criteria adds critical dimension to the evaluation.

In evaluating potential improvement actions, the team should consider the impact of the suggested improvement on organization processes, resources, and schedules. Sentinel events or near misses frequently shake up the organization's notions of the resources that should be expended in particular areas. Organizations contemplating a design or redesign effort will certainly weigh the availability of resources against the potential benefits for patients, customers, and the organization.

Asking some key questions will help the team identify the potential barriers to implementation of each potential improvement action. Relevant questions include the following:

Organization Processes

- How does the proposed action relate to other projects currently under way in the organization? Are there redundancies?
- How does the action affect other areas and processes?
- What process-related changes might be required?
- Can affected areas absorb the changes/additional responsibilities?

Resources

- What financial resources will be required to implement the action? (Include both direct and indirect costs—that is, costs associated with the necessary changes to other procedures and processes.) How will these resources be obtained?
- What other resources (staff, time, management) are required for successful implementation? How will these resources be obtained?
- What resources (capital, staff, time, management) are required for continued effectiveness? How will these resources be obtained?

Sidebar 6-2.
Evaluating Improvement Actions

- Likelihood of success (preventing recurrence or occurrence) within the organization's capabilities
- Compatibility with organization's objectives
- Risk
- Reliability
- Likelihood to engender other adverse effects
- Receptivity by management/staff/physicians
- Barriers to implementation
- Implementation time
- Long-term (versus short-term) solution
- Cost
- Measurability

Schedule

- In what time frame can implementation be completed?
- How will implementation of this action affect other schedules? How can this be handled?
- What initial and ongoing training will be required? How will this impact the schedule and how will its impact be handled?

With answers to these questions in hand, the team can better gauge whether or not the pluses outweigh the minuses.

After completing this questioning process, the team may wish to revisit the ranking exercises described previously. This can help to clarify which corrective improvement actions should be selected. To summarize the potential of each proposed action, the team can ask, "What will result from implementing this action?" and "What would result from not implementing this action?" (as shown in Worksheet 6-2, page 128).

At this point, the team should be ready to select a finite number of improvement actions. Each action must

- address a root cause;
- offer a long-term solution to the problem;
- have a greater positive than negative impact on other processes, resources, and schedules;
- be objective and measurable;
- have a clearly defined implementation time line; and
- be assignable to staff for implementation.

The next section describes how the team designs improvements and develops an action plan covering each of these aspects.

Step Fifteen: Design Improvements

The product of the root cause analysis is an action plan that identifies the strategies that the organization intends to implement to reduce the risk of similar events occurring in the future. The team is now ready to start drafting such a plan. The plan should address the five issues of what, how, when, who, and where involved in implementing and evaluating the effectiveness of proposed improvement actions.

Issue One: What
Designing *what* involves determining the scope of the actions and specific activities that will be recommended. A clear definition of the goals is critical. To understand the potential effects of the improvement activity, the organization must determine which dimension of performance—efficacy, appropriateness, availability, timeliness, effectiveness, continuity, safety, efficiency, and respect and caring—will be affected. At times, the relationship between two or more dimensions must be considered. Redesign in response to a sentinel event will most often focus on safety, but may affect any or all of the other dimensions. What specific activities will be needed to achieve the necessary improvement? Use Worksheet 6-3, page 129, to articulate responses to questions concerning goals, dimensions of performance, and required specific activities.

Issue Two: How
How does the organization expect, want, and need the improved process to perform? The team carrying out the effort should set specific expectations for

performance resulting from the design or improvement. Without these expectations, the organization will not be able to determine the degree of success of the efforts. These expectations can be derived from staff expertise, consumer expectations, experiences of other organizations, recognized standards, and other sources. What sequence of activities and resources will be required to meet these expectations? How and what will the team measure to determine whether the process is actually performing at the level expected?

The organization or group will need specific tools to measure the performance of the newly designed or improved process to determine whether expectations are met. These measures can be taken directly or adapted from other sources, or newly created, as appropriate. It is important for the measures to be as quantitative as possible. This means that the measurement can be represented by a scale or range of values. For example, if improving staff competence in calculating medication doses is cited as a corrective solution, the measure should evaluate competence before and after each training or educational session. If pretraining competence is tested at 80% to 85% proficiency, posttraining competence might be set at 90% to 95% proficiency, for example. Or, in the patient suicide example described on page 46, measures might include the percentage of accurately and appropriately completed suicide risk assessments as determined through peer review and the percentage of rooms with breakaway shower fixtures.

At times, it may be difficult to establish quantitative measures—the improvement simply seems to lend itself more to qualitative measures. Quantification of improvement is critical, however, and even when solutions can be measured only in terms of risk reduction potential, it is important to try to quantify such potential as much as possible through concrete measures.

Use Worksheet 6-4, page 130, to articulate responses to questions concerning expectations, the sequence of activities, measures, and resources required.

Issue Three: When

Next, the team must define *when* the organization must meet its improvement goals. What time frame will be established for implementing the improvement action? What time line will be established for each activity comprising the steps along the way? What are the major milestones and their respective dates? A Gantt chart of one organization's improvement plan appears as Figure 6-2, pages 114–115. Use Worksheet 6-5, page 131, to articulate responses to questions concerning time frames and milestones.

 Tool: *Gantt chart*

Issue Four: Who

Who is closest to this process and therefore should "own" the improvement activity? Who should be accountable at various stages? To a great extent, the success of an improvement effort hinges on involving the right people from all disciplines, services, and offices involved in the process being addressed. The process for taking action consists of several stages, each of which may have different players.

The group that creates the process should include the people responsible for the process, the people who will carry out the process, and the people affected by the process. As appropriate, the group members could include staff from different units, different branch offices or teams, different services, different disciplines, and different job categories. When the group needs a perspective not offered by its representatives, it should conduct interviews or surveys outside the group or invite new members into the work group. It is important to consider customers and suppliers such as purchasers, payers, physicians, referral sources, accreditors, regulators, and the community as a whole. See Worksheet 6-6, pages 132–133, for more information on key players at each stage.

Leaders and managers must take an active role in overseeing and setting priorities for design and

redesign. Generally, managers are responsible for processes within their areas; design or redesign of processes with a wider scope may be overseen by upper management or by a team of managers. Leaders must ensure that the people involved have the necessary resources and expertise. Furthermore, their authority to make changes should be commensurate with their responsibility for process improvements. While regular feedback and contact with management are important, rigid control can stifle creativity.

Issue Five: Where

Where will the improvement action be implemented? Will its implementation be organizationwide, or in a selected location, with a selected patient population or selected staff members? Are the location, target population, and target staff of the improvement action likely to expand with success? Use Worksheet 6-7, page 134, to indicate where the improvement action will be implemented. Worksheet 6-8, page 135, can be used to provide a summary look at the what, how, when, who, and where involved in implementing proposed improvement actions.

Considering the Impact of Change

When designing improvements, the team will also want to consider the impact of change on the organization. No matter how minor, improvements require change, and it is normal for individuals and organizations to resist change. Resistance to change can come from inertia, the challenge of managing the change process, the challenge of obtaining necessary knowledge to ensure that the change can be implemented effectively, and resource limitations. The team can identify areas where resistance to change might arise and plan countermeasures using Worksheet 6-9, page 136.

16 Step Sixteen: Ensure Acceptability of the Action Plan

The team has defined the what, how, when, who, and where in an improvement action plan. How does the team know whether it is acceptable to the Joint Commission as part of a root cause analysis in response to a sentinel event?

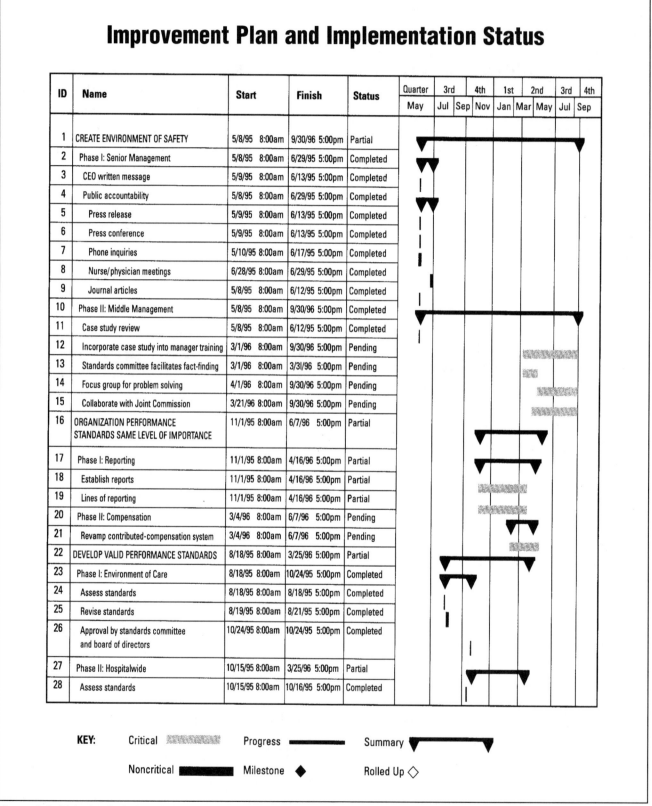

Improvement Plan and Implementation Status

ID	Name	Start	Finish	Status
1	CREATE ENVIRONMENT OF SAFETY	5/8/95 8:00am	9/30/96 5:00pm	Partial
2	Phase I: Senior Management	5/8/95 8:00am	6/29/95 5:00pm	Completed
3	CEO written message	5/9/95 8:00am	6/13/95 5:00pm	Completed
4	Public accountability	5/8/95 8:00am	6/29/95 5:00pm	Completed
5	Press release	5/9/95 8:00am	6/13/95 5:00pm	Completed
6	Press conference	5/9/95 8:00am	6/13/95 5:00pm	Completed
7	Phone inquiries	5/10/95 8:00am	6/17/95 5:00pm	Completed
8	Nurse/physician meetings	6/28/95 8:00am	6/29/95 5:00pm	Completed
9	Journal articles	5/8/95 8:00am	6/12/95 5:00pm	Completed
10	Phase II: Middle Management	5/8/95 8:00am	9/30/96 5:00pm	Completed
11	Case study review	5/8/95 8:00am	6/12/95 5:00pm	Completed
12	Incorporate case study into manager training	3/1/96 8:00am	9/30/96 5:00pm	Pending
13	Standards committee facilitates fact-finding	3/1/96 8:00am	3/3l/96 5:00pm	Pending
14	Focus group for problem solving	4/1/96 8:00am	9/30/96 5:00pm	Pending
15	Collaborate with Joint Commission	3/21/96 8:00am	9/30/96 5:00pm	Pending
16	ORGANIZATION PERFORMANCE STANDARDS SAME LEVEL OF IMPORTANCE	11/1/95 8:00am	6/7/96 5:00pm	Partial
17	Phase I: Reporting	11/1/95 8:00am	4/16/96 5:00pm	Partial
18	Establish reports	11/1/95 8:00am	4/16/96 5:00pm	Partial
19	Lines of reporting	11/1/95 8:00am	4/16/96 5:00pm	Partial
20	Phase II: Compensation	3/4/96 8:00am	6/7/96 5:00pm	Pending
21	Revamp contributed-compensation system	3/4/96 8:00am	6/7/96 5:00pm	Pending
22	DEVELOP VALID PERFORMANCE STANDARDS	8/18/95 8:00am	3/25/96 5:00pm	Partial
23	Phase I: Environment of Care	8/18/95 8:00am	10/24/95 5:00pm	Completed
24	Assess standards	8/18/95 8:00am	8/18/95 5:00pm	Completed
25	Revise standards	8/19/95 8:00am	8/21/95 5:00pm	Completed
26	Approval by standards committee and board of directors	10/24/95 8:00am	10/24/95 5:00pm	Completed
27	Phase II: Hospitalwide	10/15/95 8:00am	3/25/96 5:00pm	Partial
28	Assess standards	10/15/95 8:00am	10/16/95 5:00pm	Completed

KEY: Critical ▨▨▨ Progress ▬▬▬ Summary ▼▬▬▼

Noncritical ▬▬▬ Milestone ◆ Rolled Up ◇

Figure 6-2. This detailed plan of the steps involved in implementing the strategies, priorities, and expected time frames was created by an organization following a sentinel event involving a mechanical failure. The status of each phase in the plan is recorded so everyone involved has a clear idea of the progress being made.

Used with permission.

Improvement Plan and Implementation Status (continued)

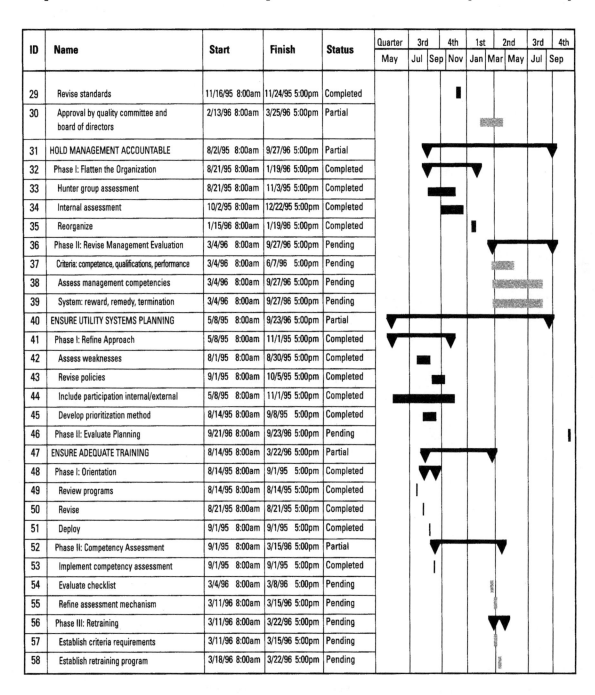

ID	Name	Start	Finish	Status	Quarter May	3rd Jul	Sep	4th Nov	1st Jan	Mar	2nd May	3rd Jul	4th Sep
29	Revise standards	11/16/95 8:00am	11/24/95 5:00pm	Completed									
30	Approval by quality committee and board of directors	2/13/96 8:00am	3/25/96 5:00pm	Partial									
31	HOLD MANAGEMENT ACCOUNTABLE	8/21/95 8:00am	9/27/96 5:00pm	Partial									
32	Phase I: Flatten the Organization	8/21/95 8:00am	1/19/96 5:00pm	Completed									
33	Hunter group assessment	8/21/95 8:00am	11/3/95 5:00pm	Completed									
34	Internal assessment	10/2/95 8:00am	12/22/95 5:00pm	Completed									
35	Reorganize	1/15/96 8:00am	1/19/96 5:00pm	Completed									
36	Phase II: Revise Management Evaluation	3/4/96 8:00am	9/27/96 5:00pm	Pending									
37	Criteria: competence, qualifications, performance	3/4/96 8:00am	6/7/96 5:00pm	Pending									
38	Assess management competencies	3/4/96 8:00am	9/27/96 5:00pm	Pending									
39	System: reward, remedy, termination	3/4/96 8:00am	9/27/96 5:00pm	Pending									
40	ENSURE UTILITY SYSTEMS PLANNING	5/8/95 8:00am	9/23/96 5:00pm	Partial									
41	Phase I: Refine Approach	5/8/95 8:00am	11/1/95 5:00pm	Completed									
42	Assess weaknesses	8/1/95 8:00am	8/30/95 5:00pm	Completed									
43	Revise policies	9/1/95 8:00am	10/5/95 5:00pm	Completed									
44	Include participation internal/external	5/8/95 8:00am	11/1/95 5:00pm	Completed									
45	Develop prioritization method	8/14/95 8:00am	9/8/95 5:00pm	Completed									
46	Phase II: Evaluate Planning	9/21/96 8:00am	9/23/96 5:00pm	Pending									
47	ENSURE ADEQUATE TRAINING	8/14/95 8:00am	3/22/96 5:00pm	Partial									
48	Phase I: Orientation	8/14/95 8:00am	9/1/95 5:00pm	Completed									
49	Review programs	8/14/95 8:00am	8/14/95 5:00pm	Completed									
50	Revise	8/21/95 8:00am	8/21/95 5:00pm	Completed									
51	Deploy	9/1/95 8:00am	9/1/95 5:00pm	Completed									
52	Phase II: Competency Assessment	9/1/95 8:00am	3/15/96 5:00pm	Partial									
53	Implement competency assessment	9/1/95 8:00am	9/1/95 5:00pm	Completed									
54	Evaluate checklist	3/4/96 8:00am	3/8/96 5:00pm	Pending									
55	Refine assessment mechanism	3/11/96 8:00am	3/15/96 5:00pm	Pending									
56	Phase III: Retraining	3/11/96 8:00am	3/22/96 5:00pm	Pending									
57	Establish criteria requirements	3/11/96 8:00am	3/15/96 5:00pm	Pending									
58	Establish retraining program	3/18/96 8:00am	3/22/96 5:00pm	Pending									

As mentioned in Chapter 1, page 15, an action plan is considered acceptable by the Joint Commission if it

- identifies changes that can be implemented to reduce risk, or formulates a rationale for not undertaking such changes; and
- where improvement actions are planned, identifies who is responsible for implementation, when the action will be implemented (including any pilot testing), and how the effectiveness of the actions will be evaluated.

Checklist 6-2, right, lists the criteria for an acceptable action plan.

17 Step Seventeen: Implement the Improvement Plan

Once the goals for improvement have been established, the organization can begin planning and carrying out the improvements. A pilot test implementing improvement on a small scale, monitoring its results, and refining the improvement actions is highly recommended. This enables the team to ensure that the improvement is successful before committing significant organization resources. Pilot testing also aids in building support for the improvement plan, thereby facilitating buy-in by opinion leaders. To pilot-test an improvement, the team will follow a systematic method that includes performing steps 18 through 21 on a limited scale.

A systematic method for design or improvement of processes can help organizations pursue identified opportunities. A standard, yet flexible, process for carrying out these changes should help leaders and others ensure that actions address root causes, involve appropriate people, and result in desired and sustained changes. Depending on an organization's mission and improvement goals, any of the processes described here may be used to implement a process improvement. Three improvement methods are described:

- The scientific method;
- The plan-do-study-act (PDSA) cycle; and
- Critical paths.

Checklist 6-2. Criteria for an Acceptable Action Plan

Check to ensure that the action plan has the following attributes:

- ☐ Identifies changes to reduce risk or provides rationale for not undertaking changes;
- ☐ Identifies who is responsible for implementation;
- ☐ Identifies when action(s) will be implemented; and
- ☐ Identifies how the effectiveness of action(s) will be evaluated.

The Scientific Method

The fundamental components of any improvement process are

- planning the change;
- testing the change;
- studying its effects; and
- implementing changes determined to be worthwhile.

Many readers will readily associate the activities listed—plan, test, study, implement—with the scientific method. Indeed, the scientific method is a fundamental, inclusive paradigm for change, and includes these steps:

- Determine what is known now (about a process, problem, topic of interest);
- Decide what needs to be learned, changed, or improved;
- Develop a hypothesis about how the change can be accomplished;
- Test the hypothesis;
- Assess the effect of the test (compare results of before versus after or traditional versus innovative); and
- Implement successful improvements or rehypothesize and conduct another experiment.

This orderly, logical, inclusive process for improvement will serve organizations well as they attempt to assess and improve performance.

The Plan-Do-Study-Act (PDSA) Cycle

A well-established process for improvement that is based on the scientific method is the PDSA cycle. (This method is also called the PDCA cycle, with the word *check* replacing the word *study*). This process is attributed to Walter Shewhart, a quality improvement pioneer with Bell Laboratories in the 1920s and 1930s, and is also widely associated with W. Edwards Deming, a student and later a colleague of Shewhart. Deming made the PDCA cycle central to his influential teachings about quality. The cycle is compelling in its logic and simplicity. A brief explanation of this process should help readers not already familiar with the cycle to understand it and its use (see Figure 6-3, page 118).

During the *planning* step, an operational plan for testing the chosen improvement action is created. Small-scale testing can help to determine whether the improvement actions are viable, whether they will have the desired result, and whether any refinements are necessary before putting them into full operation. The list of proposed improvement actions should be narrowed to a number that can be reasonably tested— perhaps between two and four, but not often more.

During the planning stage, several issues should be resolved:

- Who will be involved in the test?
- What must they know to participate in the test?
- What are the testing timetables?
- How will the test be implemented?
- Why is the idea being tested?
- What are the success factors?
- How will the process and outcomes of the test be measured and assessed?

The *do* step involves implementing the pilot test and collecting actual performance data.

During the *study* (or *check*) step, data collected during the pilot test are analyzed to determine whether the improvement action was successful in achieving the desired outcomes. To determine the degree of success, actual test performance is compared to desired performance targets and baseline results achieved using the established process.

The next step is the *act* step—to take action. If the pilot test is not successful, the cycle repeats. Once actions have been shown to be successful, they are made part of standard operating procedure. The process does not stop here. The effectiveness of the action will continue to be measured and assessed to ensure that improvement is maintained.

The components of the four-step PDSA cycle as they relate to designing and improving processes appear as Checklist 6-3, page 119. A single initiative can involve a number of different testing phases or different change strategies and can therefore require the use of consecutive PDSA cycles.

To help teams and individuals involved in design or improvement initiatives apply the method effectively, the organization, depending on the nature of the improvement project, may want to consider the questions outlined in Sidebar 6-3, page 120, at each step of the method.

Critical Paths

One type of process design or redesign that can be used in health care, particularly in response to a sentinel event in a hospital setting, is the development of a critical path (also referred to as clinical path and clinical or critical pathway). The primary objective of critical pathways is to reduce common-cause variation, thereby reducing the risk of special-cause variation (sentinel events) in dependent processes. Critical paths offer a systematic, flexible guide for standardization of patient care that can start, for example, before admission and follow the patient across all care settings. They are designed by those

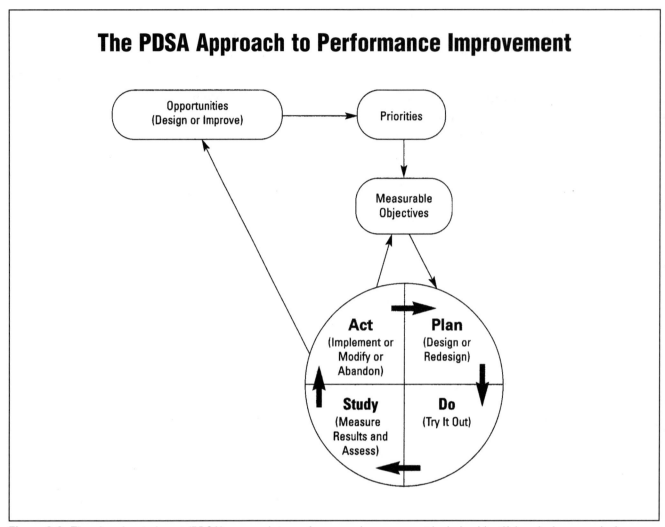

Figure 6-3. The plan-do-study-act (PDSA) approach to performance improvement includes identifying design or redesign opportunities, setting priorities for improvement, and implementing the improvement project.

involved in the process—clients, clinicians, nurses, pharmacists, and others—who come together to offer their unique perspectives and expertise.

A critical path is an excellent way to redesign an existing clinical process that needs change. One advantage of a critical path is the opportunity to start fresh, cast aside traditional but not particularly effective procedures, and research and implement the best practices. Many critical paths have been developed to date by numerous organizations, including professional societies, government agencies, and health care organizations. These may provide guidance.

A summary of the steps involved in critical path development and implementation appears as Sidebar 6-4, page 121.

Additional Improvement Tools
The following tools are useful for taking action to improve processes. For example,
- *brainstorming* can be used to create ideas for improvement actions;
- *multivoting* and *selection grids* can help a team decide among various possible improvement actions;
- *flowcharts* can help a team understand the current process and how the new or redesigned one should work;

Checklist 6-3. Components of the PDSA Cycle

Plan

- ☐ Develop or design a new process or redesign or improve an existing process.
- ☐ Determine how to test the new or redesigned process.
- ☐ Identify measures that can be used to assess the success of the strategy and whether the objective was reached.
- ☐ Determine how to collect the measures of success.
- ☐ Involve the right people in the development and testing.

Do

- ☐ Run the test of the new or redesigned process, preferably on a small scale.
- ☐ Collect data on the measures of success.

Study

- ☐ Assess the results of the test.
- ☐ Determine whether the change was successful.
- ☐ Identify any lessons learned.

Act

- ☐ Implement the change permanently;
- ☐ Modify it and run it through another testing cycle; or
- ☐ Abandon it and develop a new approach to test.

- *cause-and-effect diagrams* can indicate which changes might cause the desired result or goal;
- *Pareto charts* can help determine which changes are likely to have the greatest effect in reaching the goal;
- *run charts, control charts, line graphs, pie graphs, and scatter diagrams* can measure the effect of a process change or variation in processes and outcomes; and

- *histograms and data tables* can show how much effect each change has had.

 Tools: *Brainstorming, multivoting, selection grid, flowchart, cause-and-effect diagram, Pareto Chart, run chart, control chart, histogram, line graph, pie graphs, scatter diagram, data table*

Creating and Managing the Change

Some suggested actions the team might take to help manage and lead the change or improvement process follow.[8] These are based on eight sequential stages in the process of leading change in organizations.[9] The steps in creating and managing the change process are as follows:

1. Establish a sense of urgency by
   - identifying the "best anywhere" and the gap between one process and another,
   - identifying the consequence of being less than the best, and
   - exploring sources of complacency;
2. Create a guiding coalition to
   - find the right people,
   - create trust, and
   - share a common goal;
3. Develop a vision and strategy that is
   - easily pictured,
   - attractive,
   - feasible and clear,
   - flexible, and
   - communicable;
4. Communicate the changed vision in a way that
   - is simple,
   - uses metaphor,
   - works in multiple forms,
   - involves doing instead of telling,
   - explains inconsistencies, and
   - involves give and take;
5. Empower broad-based action by
   - communicating sensible vision to employees,
   - making organization structures compatible with action,

Sidebar 6-3. Key Questions to Consider During the PDSA Cycle

Plan
- How was a design or improvement strategy selected for testing?
- Is there knowledge-based information (for example, from the literature, other organizations, or other external sources) supporting the new or improved process?
- What issues in the external environment (such as economy, politics, customer needs, competitors, regulations) will affect the performance of the new or improved process?
- What issues in the internal environment will affect the performance of the new or improved process?
- Who is (are) the customer(s) of the process?
- What is the current process?
- What is the desired process?
- Who are the suppliers of the process?
- What changes will have the most impact?
- Is there a plan for testing the design or improvement?
- Is there a time line for testing?
- What data will be collected to determine whether the test was successful (that is, whether the objective was met)?
- How is it determined that the measures actually address the desired issue?
- Can the measures used actually track performance?
- How will data be collected?
- Who will collect data?
- Are systems in place to support planned measurement?
- Is benchmarking feasible for this initiative?
- Are the right people involved?
- What resources are needed to design or redesign the process? What resources are available?

Do
- Was the testing plan followed?
- Were needed modifications discussed with the appropriate people?
- Was data collection timely?
- Was data collection reliable?

Study
- How will the test data be assessed?
- What process should be used?
- Who should be involved in data analysis?
- What methods or tools should be used to analyze data?
- Is training needed on data analysis methods and tools?
- Is comparative data (internal or external) available?
- Does data analysis lead to an understanding of problem areas?
- Are data analysis timely? Are the results available soon enough to take needed actions?
- Did the test data indicate that the design or improvement was successful?
- What lessons were learned from the test?
- What measures will determine whether to implement the tested design or improvement on a permanent basis?
- How and to whom will the results of assessment activities be communicated?

Act
- Should changes be recommended to others (for example, for purchasing equipment or implementing specific processes)?
- How will these changes be communicated to the appropriate people?
- Is any education or training needed?
- How will gain be maintained and backsliding be prevented?
- What measures should be used to assess the performance of the new or improved product or process?
- Should any of the measures identified above be included in ongoing measurement activities?

Sidebar 6-4. Developing and Implementing a Critical Path

Selecting the Process

The initial step in creating a critical path is choosing a process to standardize. The first part of the root cause analysis will have identified the relevant process(es) that require(s) redesign. The time needed to develop a critical path may vary from two hours to four months.[1] Organizations should be prepared for a significant commitment of time.

Defining the Diagnosis, Condition, or Procedure

An appropriately defined process and patient population will simplify critical path development. A process that is too broadly defined will result in a path that is either too complex or too vague; conversely, a process that is too narrowly defined can result in a path that applies in only a limited number of cases.[2,3]

Forming a Team

The group that creates the critical path must represent all disciplines involved in the process. The scope of the process will help determine team members. Another valuable perspective comes from patients and their families or caregivers, customers, and others. The team should elicit information from the people the process is designed to benefit. Similarly, if other parties are involved but are not team members, their input must also be elicited.

Identifying or Creating the Critical Path

Team members must reach consensus on the key activities involved in each stage of the care process. Members can draw on personal experience and knowledge, existing clinical literature and practice guidelines, and patient perspectives. When varying styles or methods of care arise—as they inevitably will—the team should not panic. The resulting discussion can yield important knowledge about patient care. If varied practice patterns are such that the group cannot reach consensus, the path should not dictate one approach over the other; separate paths can be developed when necessary.[3] Subsequent outcome measurement may demonstrate an advantage of one path over the other. The path need not be limited to clinical activities; it can also include activities that surround the clinical process, such as transportation to the radiology department. Critical paths should also include descriptions of expected outcomes. Despite the complexity of the processes involved, teams should attempt to make their paths as concise as possible—one page is ideal—so they can be used as practical tools in daily practice.

Results

At all stages of the care process, organization staff can refer to critical paths. They should be available to all involved personnel in all the relevant work areas and office locations. Critical paths are also valuable for patients; they can increase patients' knowledge and sense of partnership with providers.[1-3]

References

1. Weber DO: Clinical pathways stretch patient care but shrink costly lengths of stay at Anne Arundel Medical Center in Annapolis, Maryland. *Strategic Health Excell* 5(5):1–9, 1992.
2. Bower KA: Developing and using critical paths. In Lord JT (ed): *The Physician Leader's Guide*. Rockville, MD: Bader & Associates, Inc., 1992, pp 61–66.
3. Zander K: Critical pathways. In Melum MM, Sinioris MK (eds): *Total Quality Management: The Health Care Pioneers*. Chicago: American Hospital Publishing, Inc., 1992, pp 305–314.

- providing needed training,
- aligning information and human resource systems, and
- confronting supervisors who undercut change;
6. Generate short-term wins by
   - fixing the date of certain change,
   - doing the easy stuff first, and
   - using measurement to confirm change;
7. Consolidate gains and produce more change by
   - identifying true interdependencies and smooth interconnections,
   - eliminating unnecessary dependencies, and
   - identifying linked subsequent cycles of change; and
8. Anchor new approaches in the culture with
   - results,
   - conversation,
   - turnover, and
   - succession.

18 Step Eighteen: Develop Measures of Effectiveness and Ensure Their Success

Previous pages described how to design or redesign a function or process where the improvement cycle often begins. Once a function or process is under way, the team should collect data about its performance. As described in Chapter 4, pages 78–80, measurement is the process of collecting and aggregating these data, a process that helps assess the level of performance and determine whether further improvement actions are necessary. Specifically, measurement can be used as an integral technique throughout the PDSA cycle to

- assist in process design or redesign (the *plan* step);
- test whether process design or redesign is implemented properly (the *do* step);
- assess the results of the test (the *study* step);
- provide assistance in implementing the improvement (the *act* step); and
- maintain the improvement and determine whether the improvement should be part of the organization's ongoing monitoring process (repeat of the PDSA cycle).

A description of each use appears in Chapter 4, pages 78–79. This discussion focuses on measurement's use to determine whether improvement has occurred and is sustained.

The first step in measuring the success of improvement efforts is to develop high-quality measures of effectiveness. The choice of what to measure is critical. Measurement must relate to the improvement and validate the accomplishment of the goal (or failure to do so). See Checklist 4-1, page 81, for a list of key criteria for measures, and Sidebar 4-3, page 81, for key questions the team should ask concerning what it will measure. Answer the questions in Worksheet 6-10, pages 137–138, as the team identifies, measures, and designs the measurement plan.

Some measures or performance indicators may require specific targets and these should be set by the team prior to data collection. For example, in the patient suicide case described on page 46, the team would set 100% as the target for bringing rooms in the behavioral health unit into compliance with breakaway shower fixtures. For the treatment delay example, the team would set a score of 95% as the target for all posttraining test scores. Data collection efforts should be planned and coordinated. Use a separate worksheet to plan and monitor the indicators selected to measure each improvement goal (see Worksheet 6-11, page 139). Use Checklist 6-4, page 123, to help ensure that the team has considered important attributes of measurement success.

Who should be responsible for measurement? The team, empowered to study the process and recommend changes, will usually be responsible for designing and carrying out the measurement activities necessary to determine how the process performs. After making changes to improve the process, the team should continue to apply some or all of its measures to determine whether the change has had the desired effect. Organizations may have various experts who can help design measurement activities, including experts in information management, quality improvement, and

Tip: Avoid Data Collection Redundancy
Make every effort to coordinate any ongoing measurement with data collection already taking place as part of the organization's everyday activities.

the function to be measured. The team can request its contribution on an ad hoc basis. For example, if the team is investigating a medication error and has a large amount of data to codify and process regarding the administration of a frequently ordered drug, the team may want to seek the help of information management staff with access to statistical software capable of analyzing a large volume of data.

Information management professionals and those responsible for carrying out the process being measured will be key players in data collection and analysis. The people involved will vary widely depending on the specific organization, the function being measured, and the measurement process.

19 Step Nineteen: Evaluate Implementation of Improvement Efforts

Once data are collected as part of measurement, they must be translated into information that the team can use to make judgments and draw conclusions about the performance of improvement efforts. This assessment forms the basis for further actions taken with improvement initiatives.

Numerous techniques can be used to assess the data collected. Most types of assessment require comparing data to a point of reference. These reference points may include

- internal comparisons;
- aggregate external reference databases;
- practice guidelines/parameters; and
- desired performance targets, specifications, or thresholds.

Checklist 6-4. Assuring the Success of Measurement

An affirmative answer to the following questions will give the team a good indication that it is on the right track with its efforts to measure the effectiveness of improvement initiatives.

Yes	No	
☐	☐	Is there a plan for use of the data?
☐	☐	Are the data collected reliable and valid?
☐	☐	Has ease of data collection been assured?
☐	☐	Have key elements required for improvement been defined?
☐	☐	Has a "data rich/information poor" syndrome been avoided?
☐	☐	Has a key point for information dissemination been designated?

Internal Comparisons

The team can compare its current performance with its past performance using statistical quality control tools. Three such tools are especially helpful in comparing performance with historical patterns and assessing variation and stability: run charts, control charts, and histograms. These show changes over time, variation in performance, and the stability of performance.

Tools: *Run chart, control chart, histogram*

Aggregate External Reference Databases

In addition to assessing the organization's own

historical patterns of performance, the team can compare the organization's performance with that of other organizations. Expanding the scope of comparison helps an organization draw conclusions about its own performance and learn about different methods to design and carry out processes. Aggregate external databases take various forms. Aggregate, risk-adjusted data about specific indicators help each organization set priorities for improvement by showing whether its current performance falls within the expected range.

One method of comparing performance is benchmarking. Although a benchmark can be any point of comparison, most often it is a standard of excellence. *Benchmarking* is the process by which one organization studies the exemplary performance of a similar process in another organization and, to the greatest extent possible, adapts that information for its own use. Or the team may wish to simply compare its results with those of other organizations or with current research or literature.

Assessment is not confined to information gathered within the walls of a single organization. To better understand its level of performance, an organization will want to compare its performance against reference databases, professional standards, trade association guidelines, and other sources.

Practice Guidelines or Parameters

Practice guidelines or parameters, critical paths, and other standardized patient care procedures are very useful reference points for comparison. Whether developed by professional societies or in-house practitioners, these procedures represent an expert consensus about the expected practices for a given diagnosis or treatment. Assessing variation from such established procedures can help the team identify how to improve a process.

Desired Performance Targets

The team may also establish targets, specifications, or thresholds for evaluation against which the

organization compares current performance. Such levels can be derived from professional literature or expert opinion within the organization.

20 Step Twenty: Take Additional Action

The team's assessment of the data collected will indicate whether or not the organization is achieving established targets or goals. If it is achieving the goals, the team's efforts now should focus on communicating, standardizing, and "rolling out" the successful improvement initiatives. The team can

- communicate the results, as described in step 21, pages 124–126;
- revise processes and procedures so that the improvement is realized in everyday work;
- complete necessary training so that all staff are up to speed on the new process or procedure;
- establish a plan to monitor the improvement's ongoing effectiveness; and
- identify other areas where the improvement could be "rolled out."

Organizations frequently falter when continued measurement indicates that improvement goals are not being sustained. Efforts tend, more often than not, to provide short-term rather than long-term improvement. If the team is not achieving the improvement goals, it will need to revisit the improvement actions by circling back to confirm root causes, identify a risk reduction strategy, design an improvement, implement an action plan, and measure the effectiveness of that plan over time.

There are a number of reasons why a team's improvements may falter and fail.[10] If the team is having trouble effecting improvement, consider the reasons and remedies shown in Sidebar 6-5, page 125.

21 Step Twenty-one: Communicate the Results

Throughout the root cause analysis process, the team should be communicating team conclusions and recommendations as outlined by the team early in the process (see Chapter 3, pages 55 and 57). Hence,

Sidebar 6-5. When Improvements Falter: Reasons and Remedies

Problem

- Failure to hold the gains because the improvement required major changes.
- Failure to hold the gains because the improvement created extra work or hassle.
- Failure to hold the gains because new staff or leadership were not trained in the improved process.
- Inability to replicate in other settings.
- Not enough public or personal attention to improvement success.
- Inadequate institutional and administrative support.
- Hidden barriers to needed changes.
- A cookie-cutter approach to replicating improvement.

Remedy

- Big changes are best arrived at one step at a time.
- Design improvements so the desired task is the easiest thing to be done. Design a robust process that makes it easy to do things right and difficult to do things incorrectly.

- Ensure continued training of all appropriate staff.
- Build a lasting improvement by recognizing that individuals adopt innovations after passing through a series of stages, including knowledge (becoming aware that a new idea exists), persuasion (forming a favorable attitude toward the new idea), decision (choosing to adopt the innovation), implementation (putting the idea into use), and confirmation (seeking further confirmation about the innovation leading to either continued adoption or discontinuance). Consider and plan for this process when bringing this improvement to each and every setting.
- Leaders must ensure that improvement successes are recognized and celebrated.
- Leaders must provide time and talent.
- Leaders must empower improvement teams to identify where changes are needed and help them make the changes happen.
- Process improvements must be reinvented at each new site, adapted to meet local circumstances, and fingerprinted by the local owners of the newly improved process.

Source: James BC, Ryer J: Holding the gains. In Nelson EC, Batalden PB, Ryer J (eds): *Clinical Improvement Action Guide.* Oakbrook Terrace, IL: Joint Commission on Accreditation of Healthcare Organizations, 1998, pp 121–124.

the communication process occurs throughout the team's effort and is critical to the success of improvement initiatives.

After determining what happened or could have happened and identifying root causes of the event or possible event, the team should provide leadership with the recommendations for improvement actions to prevent a recurrence of the event. Generally, a short

written report will provide leaders with the summary they need. An outline of the contents of such a report appears as Sidebar 6-6, page 126. The team will want to consider with care how and to whom the report is to be presented. Participants during a formal oral presentation should include those whose approval and help is needed, as well as those who could gain from the team's recommendations. Consider the following questions in communicating an improvement initiative:

Sidebar 6-6. Possible Content of Report to Leaders

Event Description

This section includes a brief description of the sentinel event or possible event. It includes what, when, where, who, and how information is articulated in the problem definition (see Chapter 3, pages 50–52). The emphasis is on facts related to the event and the areas involved.

Scope of Analysis

This section describes the team's membership and purpose, and the analytical methods used to investigate the event or possible event.

Proximate Causes and Immediate Responses

This section describes the circumstances leading to the event, proximate causes identified by the team, and any response strategies and corrective actions implemented by individuals immediately following the event.

Root Causes

This section describes the analyses conducted to determine root causes and lists the root causes identified by the team.

Improvement Actions and Follow-up Plan

This section describes the improvement actions recommended by the team for each root cause. It also describes the measures and time frame recommended to evaluate the effectiveness of improvement actions.

Following implementation of such actions and measuring and assuring their success, the team should report to leadership on the results of the improvement actions. The report should include information regarding applicability to other processes, areas, and locations, and the lessons learned.

References

1. Leape LL: Error in medicine. *JAMA* 272(23):1855, 1994.
2. Moray N: Error reduction as a systems problem. In Bogner MS (ed): *Human Error in Medicine*. Hillsdale, NJ: Lawrence Erlbaum Associates, 1994, pp 70–71.
3. Leape, p 1854.
4. Joint Commission Resources. *Failure Mode and Effects Analysis (FMEA): Proactive Risk Reduction*. Oakbrook Terrace, IL: 2002.
5. Fletcher CE: Failure mode and effects analysis: An interdisciplinary way to analyze and reduce medication errors. *J Nurs Adm* 27(12):19–26, 1997.
6. Wilson PF, Dell LD, Anderson GF: *Root Cause Analysis: A Tool for Total Quality Management*. Milwaukee: ASQC Quality Press, 1993, p 75.
7. Ammerman M: *The Root Cause Analysis Handbook: A Simplified Approach to Identifying, Correcting, and Reporting Workplace Errors*. New York: Quality Resources, 1998, p 73.
8. Nelson EC, Batalden PB, Ryer J (eds): *Clinical Improvement Action Guide*. Oakbrook Terrace, IL: Joint Commission, 1998, pp 116–117.
9. Kotter JP: *Leading Change*. Boston: Harvard Business School Press, 1996.
10. James BC, Ryer J: Holding the gains: building durable improvements into everyday care delivery. In Nelson, Batalden, Ryer, pp 121–124.

- How will implementation of this initiative be communicated throughout the organization? Who needs to know?
- What communication vehicles will the team use for various audiences (individuals both directly and indirectly affected by the improvement)?

Worksheet 6-1. Prioritizing Improvement Actions

Use this worksheet to catalog improvement actions suggested by the team. Separate sheets for each root cause and its suggested improvement actions may be used. The team will also want to rate or rank improvement actions based on agreed-upon criteria. Use this worksheet to record the rankings of individual team members and the team as a whole.

Root Causes   **Suggested Improvement Actions**   **Ranking**

Root Cause 1: _____   _____   _____

_____   _____   _____

_____   _____   _____

_____   _____   _____

_____   _____   _____

Root Cause 2: _____   _____   _____

_____   _____   _____

_____   _____   _____

_____   _____   _____

_____   _____   _____

Root Cause 3: _____   _____   _____

_____   _____   _____

_____   _____   _____

_____   _____   _____

_____   _____   _____

Worksheet 6-2. Summarizing the Potential of Improvement Actions

Two questions will help the team to summarize the potential of each proposed improvement action. Use this space to provide a concise answer to each.

What will result from implementing this action?

_____

_____

_____

_____

_____

_____

_____

What would result from not implementing this action?

_____

_____

_____

_____

_____

_____

_____

Worksheet 6-3. Defining Improvement Goals, Scope, and Activities

This worksheet will help the team define what it is trying to improve. Use the space below each question to provide as concise an answer as possible.

What goals does the organization have in implementing necessary improvements related to a sentinel event or possible event?

_____

_____

_____

_____

What dimensions of performance will be most affected by the change?

_____

_____

_____

_____

What specific activities must be carried out to reach the goals and affect the dimensions of performance? (Provide a clear statement of the essential features of each proposed solution.) What are the sequential steps necessary to accomplish the proposed improvement?

1. _____

2. _____

3. _____

4. _____

5. _____

6. _____

Worksheet 6-4. Defining Improvement Expectations, Sequence, Resources, and Measures

This worksheet will help the team define how the organization will meet its improvement goals. Use the space below each question to provide as concise an answer as possible.

How must the improved process perform?

_____

_____

_____

What sequence of activities will be required to meet these expectations?

_____

_____

_____

What resources will be required to meet these expectations?

_____

_____

_____

How and what will be measured to determine whether the process is actually performing at the level expected?

Improvement Action   **Quantitative Measure**

_____

_____

_____

_____

_____

Worksheet 6-5. Defining Time Frames and Milestones

This worksheet will help the team define when the organization will meet its improvement goals. Use the space below each question to provide as concise an answer as possible.

What time frame will be established for implementing the overall improvement action?

_____

_____

_____

_____

_____

What time line will be established for each activity comprising the steps along the way?

Activity   **Time frame**

_____

_____

_____

_____

_____

What are the major milestones and their respective completion dates?

Milestone   **Completion date**

_____

_____

_____

_____

_____

Worksheet 6-6. Involving the Right People

Involving the right people at each stage of the improvement process is critical to the success of the improvement initiative. Consider which individuals should be involved at each stage and write their names in the appropriate spaces.

Designing the action. In general, the group that participated in the root cause analysis should have the necessary expertise to recommend improvements and may be in the best position to design or redesign the improvements. This group should include those who carry out or are affected by the process. They are

_____

_____

_____

_____

_____

_____

Approving recommended actions. When substantial resources are involved and the potential effects are significant, the organization's leaders will usually have to approve the action. This will most certainly be the case with improvements recommended following a sentinel event. If a group has obtained the necessary input and buy-in while devising an improvement, the approval should come readily. The appropriate leaders are

_____

_____

_____

_____

_____

_____

Worksheet 6-6. Involving the Right People (continued)

Testing the action. Testing should occur under "real world" conditions, involving staff who will actually be carrying out the process. Effects can be measured with the same methods used to establish a performance baseline. Appropriate staff members include

_____

_____

_____

_____

_____

_____

_____

Implementing the action. Although full-scale implementation of a process change should have positive results, any change can create anxiety. Therefore, care should be taken to prepare people for change and to explain the reason for the change in an educational, nonthreatening way. Cooperation is essential for changes to succeed, but will not occur if people believe a change is being forced on them without good reason. An effective team should have already acquired much of the necessary buy-in during earlier phases of the improvement process or during the early stages in the root cause analysis. Appropriate staff members include

_____

_____

_____

_____

_____

_____

_____

Worksheet 6-7. Determining Location of Improvement Actions

This worksheet will help the team define where the organization will implement improvement goals.

Where will the improvement action be implemented?

_____

_____

_____

_____

_____

Will its implementation be organizationwide, or in a selected location, with a selected patient population or selected staff members?

_____

_____

_____

_____

_____

Are the location, target population, and target staff of the improvement action likely to expand with success?

       ☐ No (If no, why not?)   ☐ Yes (If yes, how?)

_____

_____

_____

_____

_____

Worksheet 6-8. Integrating the Improvement Plan

Define the time lines and responsibilities associated with each of the project steps using the following table (customize column headers as desired). Questions to consider include the following:

- What are the time lines for each step of the project and for the project as a whole?
- What will be the checkpoints, control points, or milestones for project assessment?
- Who is responsible for each step or milestone?
- Who is responsible for corrective course action?
- Which staff members will be involved in the improvement project?
- What will be the nature and extent of their responsibilities?

Steps to Be Taken	Date of Implementation	Areas for Implementation	Individuals Responsible	Other Considerations

Worksheet 6-9. Identifying Change Barriers and Solutions

Use this worksheet to identify possible barriers to change and solutions to overcome such barriers.

Areas where resistance to change might emerge include

_____

_____

_____

_____

_____

_____

_____

_____

Countermeasures to overcome such barriers include

_____

_____

_____

_____

_____

_____

_____

_____

_____

_____

Worksheet 6-10. Designing the Measurement Plan

What is the scope of measurement for the improvement project?

_____

_____

Have any portions of the process under study been measured in the past? If so, are assessments available?

_____

_____

What measurement tools will be used for this initiative?

_____

_____

Will the tools provide reliable data? Have they been tested?

_____

_____

What costs are associated with collecting the necessary data? Do benefits outweigh costs?

_____

_____

Can the data generated by the selected measurement tool be transformed into meaningful and useful information?

_____

_____

How does the team ensure that the data are complete, accurate, and unbiased?

_____

_____

Worksheet 6-10. Designing the Measurement Plan (continued)

How will the staff collecting data be educated?

_____

_____

_____

_____

What format(s) will be used to report the data?

_____

_____

_____

_____

Where and how will any additional data needed be obtained?

_____

_____

_____

_____

How will the success of the improvement be measured?

_____

_____

_____

_____

Source: Adapted from Hanold LS, Vinson BE, Rubino A: Evaluating and improving the medication use system. In Cousins DD (ed): *Medication Use: A Systems Approach to Reducing Errors*. Oakbrook Terrace, IL: Joint Commission on Accreditation of Healthcare Organizations, 1998, pp 93–96.

Worksheet 6-11. Evaluating Target Goals

Use a worksheet like this one to plan and monitor progress in measuring the effectiveness of each improvement goal.

Goal	Measure	Person Responsible	Review Completed

Chapter 7
Tools and Techniques

This chapter provides information on selected tools and techniques that can be used during root cause analysis. The tools and techniques are presented in a uniform profile, to assist readers with their selection and use. *Profiles* identify the stage during which the tool or technique may be used, its purpose, simple usage steps, and tips for effective use. An example of the tool or technique follows.

When embarking on a root cause analysis, team members may wish to start by consulting the tool matrix appearing as Figure 7-1, page 142. This matrix lists many of the tools and techniques available during root cause analysis and indicates the stages during which they may be particularly helpful. Not all of the tools listed in the matrix are profiled in this chapter. For additional information on specific tools and techniques, readers are advised to consult the Selected Bibliography, which contains references to many excellent monographs and workbooks.

Tool Profile:
Affinity diagram
(See Figure 7-2, page 143.)

Stage to Use: Identifying proximate causes; identifying root causes; identifying improvement opportunities.

Purpose: To creatively generate a large volume of ideas or issues and then organize them into meaningful groups.

Simple Steps to Success:
1. Choose a team.
2. Define the issue in the broadest and most neutral manner.
3. Brainstorm the issue and record the ideas.
4. Randomly display cards or notes with the ideas so that everyone can see them.
5. Sort the ideas into groups of related topics.
6. Create header or title cards for each grouping.
7. Draw the diagram, connecting all header cards with their groupings.

Tips for Effective Use
- Keep the team small (four to six people) and ensure varied perspectives.
- Generate as many ideas as possible using brainstorming guidelines.
- Record ideas from brainstorming on index cards or adhesive notes.
- Sort the ideas in silence, being guided in sorting only by gut instinct.
- If an idea keeps getting moved back and forth from one group to another, agree to create a duplicate card or note.
- Reach a consensus on how cards are sorted.
- Allow for some ideas to stand alone.
- Make sure that each idea has at least a noun and a verb when appropriate; avoid using single words. (See others to follow)
- Break large groupings into subgroups with subtitles, but be careful not to slow progress with too much definition.

Tool Matrix

Tools	Proximate	Root	Identifying Improvements	Implementing and Monitoring Improvements
Affinity diagram	x	x	x	
Barrier analysis	x			x
Box plot		x		
Brainstorming	x		x	
Cause-and-effect diagram	x	x		
Change analysis	x			
Checksheets		x		x
Contingency diagram	x		x	x
Control charts		x	x	x
Cost-of-quality analysis	x			
Critical-to-quality analysis	x			
Decision matrix		x	x	
Deployment flowchart	x		x	x
Effective-achievable matrix		x	x	
Failure mode and effects analysis			x	
Fault tree analysis	x	x	x	
Fishbone diagram	x	x		
Flowchart	x	x	x	x
Force field analysis	x		x	x
Gantt chart	x	x	x	x
Graphs		x		x
Histogram	x	x	x	x
Ishikawa diagram	x	x		
Is–Is not matrix		x		
Kolmogorov-Smirnov test		x		x
List reduction		x	x	
Matrix diagram		x	x	x
Multivoting	x	x	x	
Nominal group technique (NGT)	x		x	
Normal probability plot		x		x
Operational definitions		x	x	x
Pareto chart		x	x	
PDSA (plan-do-study-act) cycle				x
PMI (plus, minus, interesting)		x	x	
Relations diagram	x	x	x	
Run chart	x	x		x
Scatter diagram (scattergram)		x		x
Storyboard			x	x
Stratification		x		
Time line	x	x		
Top-down flowchart	x		x	x
Why-why diagram	x			
Work-flow diagram	x		x	x

Figure 7-1. This matrix lists many of the tools and techniques available during root cause analysis and indicates the stages during which they may be particularly helpful. Not all of the tools are profiled in this chapter.

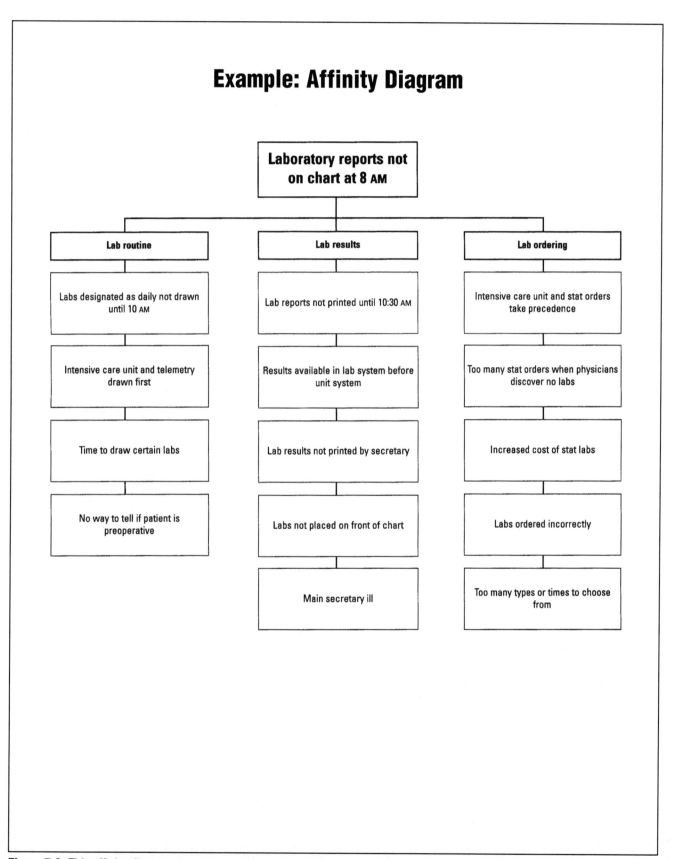

Figure 7-2. This affinity diagram shows how a wide range of ideas can be arranged in manageable order. Using this type of diagram presents ideas on why laboratory results are not available as needed into three categories: routine, results, and ordering.

Tool Profile:
Barrier analysis
(See Figure 7-3, page 145.)

Stage to Use: Identifying proximate causes; implementing and monitoring improvements.

Purpose: To offer a structured way to visualize the events related to system failure or the creation of a problem. It can be used reactively to solve problems, investigate sentinel events, or identify missing safeguards, or proactively to evaluate existing barriers or identify additional barriers that should be considered to prevent recurrence of unwanted events.

Simple Steps to Success:
1. Define the targets. *Targets* are those things of value that can be harmed by threats. Identify what has been damaged or could have been damaged by the threat.
2. Identify the threat. *Threats* are those hazards or potential problems that cause harm or an adverse outcome or have the potential to do so.
3. Identify the barriers. *Barriers* are those things that should have prevented or could prevent the undesired event.
4. Analyze the barriers. This involves analyzing the adequacy of the barriers by asking questions about their performance.
5. Identify apparent or proximate causes and the root causes. List all the proximate causes and root cause(s).
6. Devise and recommend corrective or preventive actions.

Tips for Effective Use
- Remember that the list of targets may include multiple items.
- Be aware that with sentinel events occurring in health care facilities, targets are generally the people, either individually or collectively, who can be damaged or harmed by an unwanted incident. However, targets can also be material things such as buildings and equipment; nonmaterial things such as goodwill, friendship, and status; or the environment.
- List all the potential targets initially and let follow-up analysis eliminate those not affected by the event.
- To analyze the barriers, ask the questions, "Were barriers in place to minimize threats to the target? Were such barriers adequate? That is, were they capable of handling the threat? Were there backups for each barrier?"
- Be aware that each less-than-adequate barrier can be attributed to a different proximate cause.
- The root cause can be identified as the cause that appears most often in explaining inadequate barriers, or the cause that, if eliminated, would preclude the event from happening.
- Use a simple worksheet to record the barrier analysis.

Example: Generic Barrier Analysis Worksheet

Target	Threat	Barrier	Analysis

Figure 7-3. This generic worksheet shows a simple way of listing and comparing information for barrier analysis. The worksheet is arranged in columns to lead logically from the target to threat(s), barrier(s), and analysis.

Source: Wilson PF, Dell LD, Anderson GF: *Root Cause Analysis: A Tool for Total Quality Management*. Milwaukee: ASQC Quality Press, 1993, p 147. Used with permission.

Tool Profile:
Brainstorming
(See Figure 7-4, page 147.)

Stage to Use: Identifying proximate causes; identifying improvement opportunities.

Purpose: To generate multiple ideas in a minimum amount of time through a creative group process.

Simple Steps to Success:

1. Define the subject. This ensures that the session will have direction.
2. Think briefly about the issue. Allow enough time for team members to gather their thoughts, but not enough time for detailed analysis.
3. Set a time limit. There should be enough time for every member to make a contribution, but keep it short to prevent premature analysis of ideas.
4. Generate ideas. Use a structured format in which the group members express ideas by taking turns in a predetermined order and the process continues in rotation until either time runs out or ideas are exhausted. Or, use an unstructured format in which group members voice ideas as they come to mind.
5. Clarify ideas. The goal is to make sure that all ideas are recorded accurately and are understood by the group.

Tips for Effective Use

- Create a nonthreatening, safe environment for expressing ideas.
- Tell the group up front that any idea is welcome, no matter how narrow or broad in scope, how serious or light in nature. All ideas are valuable, as long as they address the subject at hand.
- Remember that the best ideas are sometimes the most unusual.
- Never criticize ideas. It is crucial that neither the leader nor the other group members comment on any given idea.
- In thinking briefly about the issue (step 2), do not give group members time to second-guess their ideas. Be aware that self-censorship will stifle creative thought.
- Write down all ideas on a chalkboard or easel so that the group can view them.
- Keep it short; enforce a time limit of 10 to 20 minutes.
- In organizations where staff may not regularly be in a centralized location, brainstorming can be done by asking staff to submit as many ideas as possible about the topic in writing, by voice mail, or by electronic mail.
- Limit brainstorming to one "level" at a time. For example, when brainstorming possible causes of miscommunication of patient information identified as contributing to the proximate cause of a medication error, teams should hold off on exploring deeper causes such as organization culture and leadership issues.
- Note deeper root causes that emerge during brainstorming in a "parking lot" list for consideration later.

Example: Brainstorming List

Possible causes of a surgical error include the following:

- No timely case review;
- No mechanism to ensure patient identity;
- Informal case referral process;
- Untimely operative dictation;
- Inadequate presurgical evaluation;
- No review of patient care information prior to surgery;
- Inadequate informed consent;
- Patient care information unavailable for preoperative review;

- Failure to perform surgery in a safe manner;
- Laterality not clearly identified;
- Delay in reporting of incident;
- No multidisciplinary review;
- Ignored pathology reports;
- History of inadequate documentation in medical record;
- Procedures performed without adequate expertise;
- Failure to take responsibility for actions; and
- No surgical plan/preoperative findings.

Figure 7-4. This figure shows an excerpt from a list one organization created using brainstorming to identify possible causes of a surgical error. This list was used to create the cause-and-effect diagram appearing as Figure 7-5, page 149. As the example shows, the ideas are widely varied, and some seem more viable than others. This is intended: Brainstorming is for generating ideas, not sorting or judging them.

Tool Profile:
Cause-and-effect diagram (Synonyms: fishbone diagram, Ishikawa diagram)
(See Figure 7-5, page 149.)

Stage to Use: Identifying proximate causes; identifying root causes.

Purpose: To present a clear picture of the many causal relationships between outcomes and the contributing factors in those outcomes.

Simple Steps to Success:
1. Identify the outcome or problem statement.
2. Determine general categories for the causes.
3. List proximate causes under each general category.
4. List underlying causes related to each proximate cause.
5. Evaluate the diagram.

Tips for Effective Use
- Make sure everyone agrees on the problem statement or outcome.
- Be succinct and stay within the team's realm of control.
- Place the outcome on the right side of the page, halfway down, and then, from the left, draw an arrow horizontally across the page, pointing to the outcome.
- Represent common categories, including work methods, personnel, materials, and equipment, on the diagram by connecting them with diagonal lines branching off from the main horizontal line.
- Brainstorm to come up with the important proximate causes. Place each proximate cause on a horizontal line connected to the appropriate diagonal line.
- Gather data to determine the relative frequencies of the causes.
- Look for causes that appear continually in the evaluation process.
- Keep asking "Why?" to reach the root cause.
- Focus on system causes, not on causes associated with individual performance.

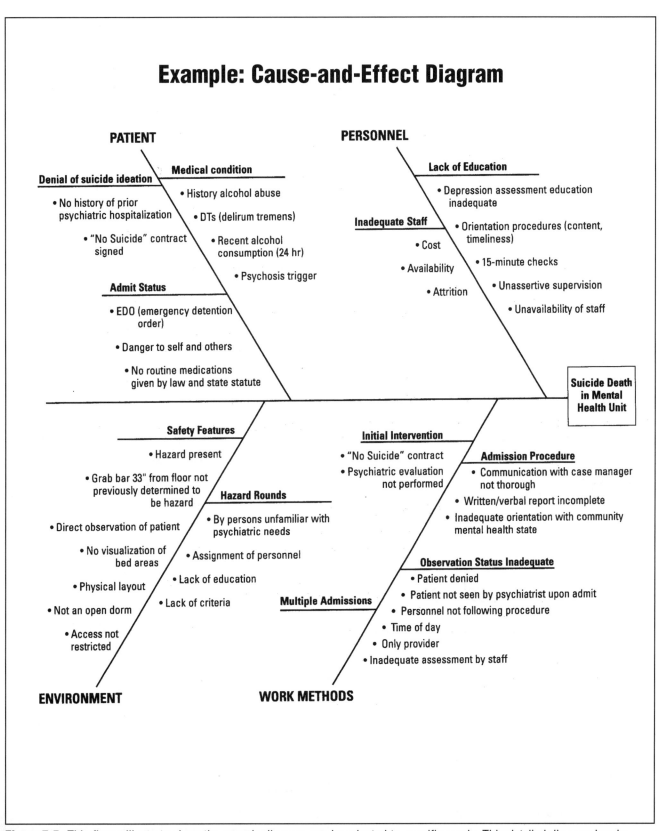

Example: Cause-and-Effect Diagram

PATIENT

Denial of suicide ideation
- No history of prior psychiatric hospitalization
- "No Suicide" contract signed

Medical condition
- History alcohol abuse
- DTs (delirum tremens)
- Recent alcohol consumption (24 hr)
- Psychosis trigger

Admit Status
- EDO (emergency detention order)
- Danger to self and others
- No routine medications given by law and state statute

PERSONNEL

Lack of Education
- Depression assessment education inadequate
- Orientation procedures (content, timeliness)
- 15-minute checks
- Unassertive supervision
- Unavailability of staff

Inadequate Staff
- Cost
- Availability
- Attrition

Safety Features
- Hazard present
- Grab bar 33" from floor not previously determined to be hazard
- Direct observation of patient
- No visualization of bed areas
- Physical layout
- Not an open dorm
- Access not restricted

Hazard Rounds
- By persons unfamiliar with psychiatric needs
- Assignment of personnel
- Lack of education
- Lack of criteria

Multiple Admissions

Initial Intervention
- "No Suicide" contract
- Psychiatric evaluation not performed

Admission Procedure
- Communication with case manager not thorough
- Written/verbal report incomplete
- Inadequate orientation with community mental health state

Observation Status Inadequate
- Patient denied
- Patient not seen by psychiatrist upon admit
- Personnel not following procedure
- Time of day
- Only provider
- Inadequate assessment by staff

ENVIRONMENT

WORK METHODS

Suicide Death in Mental Health Unit

Figure 7-5. This figure illustrates how the generic diagram can be adapted to specific needs. This detailed diagram breaks down the contributory factors that led to a sentinel event—the suicide of a patient in a mental health unit. By analyzing the proximate and underlying causes listed, staff members can identify and prioritize areas for improvement.
Used with permission.

Tool Profile:
Change analysis
(See Figure 7-6, below.)

Stage to Use: Identifying proximate causes; identifying root causes.

Purpose: To determine the proximate and root cause(s) of an event by examining the effects of change. This involves identifying all changes, either perceived or observed, and all the possible factors related to the changes.

Simple Steps to Success:
1. Identify the problem, situation, or sentinel event.
2. Describe an event-free or no-problem situation. Try to describe the situation without problems in as much detail as possible. Include the who, what, where, when, and how information listed in step 1.
3. Compare the two. Take a close look at the event and nonevent descriptions and try to detect how these situations differ.
4. List all the differences.
5. Analyze the differences. Carefully assess the differences and identify possible underlying causes.

Tips for Effective Use
- Describe the problem as accurately and in as much detail as possible. Include in the description who was involved, what was involved, where the event took place, when it took place, and what might have been a factor in causing the event.
- Once a change analysis is performed, additional questions must be asked to determine how the changes were allowed to happen.
- Continue the questioning process into the organization's systems.
- Remember that not all changes create problems; rather, change can be viewed as a force that can either positively or negatively affect the way a system, process, or individual functions.

Describe how these affected the event. Did each difference or change explain the result?
6. Integrate information and specify root cause(s). Identify the cause that, if eliminated, would have led to a nonevent situation.

Example: Change Analysis Worksheet

Event	Nonevent	Differences	Analysis

Figure 7-6. This generic worksheet shows a simple way of listing and comparing information for change analysis. The worksheet is arranged in columns to lead logically to from "what happened and what did not happen, to the differences between them, and an analysis".

Tool Profile:
Control chart
(See Figure 7-7, page 152.)

Stage to Use: Identifying root causes; identifying opportunities for improvement; implementing and monitoring improvements.

Purpose: To identify the type of variation in a process and whether the process is statistically in control.

Simple Steps to Success:

1. Choose a process to evaluate and obtain a data set.
2. Calculate the average.
3. Calculate the standard deviation. The standard deviation is a measure of the data set's variability; it is equal to the square root of the mean of all the squares of the deviations of the mean.
4. Set upper and lower control limits. Control limits should be three times higher or lower than the standard deviation relative to the mean.
5. Create the control chart. In creating the control chart, plot the mean (that is, center line) and the upper and lower control limits.
6. Plot the data points for each point in time and connect them with a line.
7. Analyze the chart and investigate findings.

Tips for Effective Use

- Obtain data before making any adjustments to the process.
- In plotting data points, keep the data in the same sequence in which they were collected.
- Be aware that special causes of variation must be eliminated before the process can be fundamentally improved and before the control chart can be used as a monitoring tool.
- Some special causes of variation are planned changes to improve the process. If the special cause is moving in the right direction toward improvement, retain the plan. It is working.
- The terms *in control* and *out of control* do not signify whether a process meets the desired level of performance. A process may be in control but consistently poor in terms of quality, and the reverse may be true.
- Charting something accomplishes nothing; it must be followed by investigation and appropriate action.
- Processes as a rule are not static. Any change can alter the process distribution and should trigger recalculation of control limits once the process change is permanently maintained and sustained (that is, greater than 8 to 12 points on one side of the process mean [center line]).
- Four rules to identify out of control processes are
  - one point on the chart is beyond three standard deviations of the mean;
  - two of three consecutive data points are on the same side of the mean and are beyond two standard deviations of the mean;
  - four of five consecutive data points are on the same side of the mean and are beyond one standard deviation of the mean; and
  - eight data points are on one side of the mean.

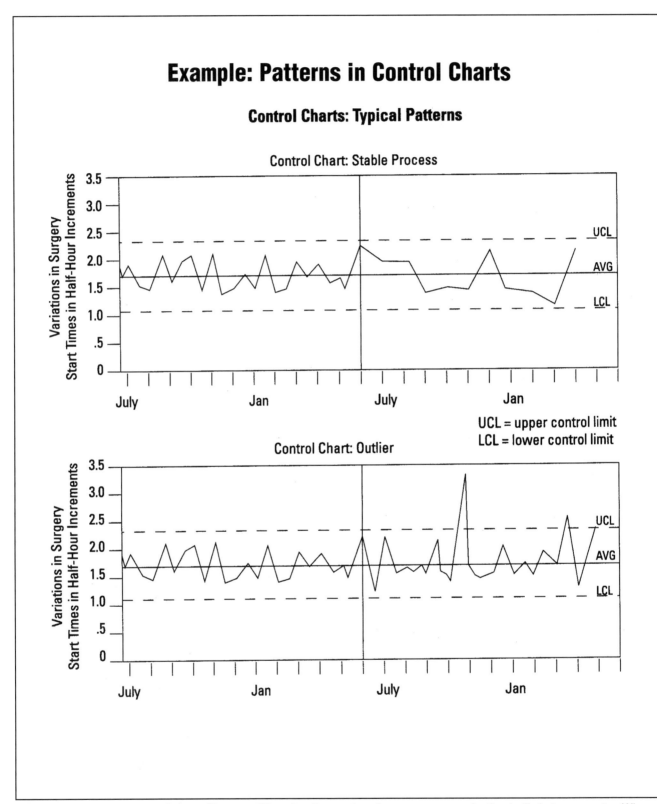

Example: Patterns in Control Charts

Control Charts: Typical Patterns

Control Chart: Stable Process

UCL = upper control limit
LCL = lower control limit

Control Chart: Outlier

Figure 7-7. These two control charts illustrate different patterns of performance an organization is likely to encounter. When performance is said to be "in control" (top chart), it does not mean desirable; rather, it means a process is stable, not affected by special causes of variation (such as equipment failure). A process should be in control before it can be systematically improved. When one point jumps outside a control limit, it is said to be an outlier (bottom chart). Staff should determine whether this single occurrence is likely to recur.

Tool Profile:

Failure mode and effects analysis (FMEA) (Synonym: failure mode, effects, and criticality analysis)
(See Figure 7-8, page 154.)

Stage to Use: Identifying opportunities for improvement.

Purpose: To examine a prospective design for possible ways in which failure can occur so that actions can be taken to eliminate the possibility of failure, stop a failure before it reaches people, or minimize the consequences of a failure.

Simple Steps to Success:

- Select a high-risk process and assemble a team.
- Diagram the process.
- Brainstorm potential failure modes and determine their effects.
- Prioritize failure modes (often accomplished through calculating a risk priority number).
- Find root causes of failure modes.
- Redesign the process.
- Analyze and test the new process.
- Implement and monitor the redesigned process.

Tips for Effective Use

- Risk priority numbers may be calculated as the product of ratings on frequency of occurrence, severity, and likelihood of detection.
- Remember that this type of analysis is generally proactive (used before an adverse event occurs), although use during root cause analyses to formulate and evaluate improvement actions is also recommended and described in this publication on page 104.

Example: Process for Failure Mode and Effects Analysis

① Item _____   ② Analysis Engineer _____

                                                   Date _____

③ Function _____

Mode of Failure	Mechanism and Cause of Failure	Effects of Failure	Frequency of Occurrence	Degree of Severity	Chance of Direction
④	⑤	⑥	⑦	⑧	⑨

Risk Priority Number	Design Action	Design Validation
⑩ = ⑦ × ⑧ × ⑨	⑪	⑫

Failure Mode and Effects Analysis Form Entry Explanation

1. Item—Item to which analysis applies.
2. Analysis Engineer—An engineer in charge of design project.
3. Function—Function of the item as user perceives it. This description should be as broad as possible.
4. Mode of Failure—A mode in which the item will fail as perceived by user.
5. Mechanism and Cause of Failure—What causes failure to occur?
6. Effects of Failure—What effects will this failure have on the user or nearby person or nearby property?
7. Frequency of Occurrence (1–10)—How often is this failure expected to occur? This column is subjectively rated on a 1 to 10 basis.
   - 1 = Rare occurrence
   - 10 = Almost certain occurrence
8. Degree of Severity (1–10)—How severe is the effect of this failure on the user or anything else? This column is subjectively rated on a 1 to 10 basis.
   - 1 = Insignificant loss to user
   - 10 = Product inoperable or major replacement cost or safety hazard
9. Degree of Detection (1–10)—Can problem be detected by the user before it does the damage? This column is subjectively rated on a 1 to 10 basis.
   - 1 = Certain detection before failure
   - 10 = No detection possible before failure
10. Risk Priority Number (1–1,000)—Order of problem-solving priority is given by multiplying numbers in columns 7, 8, and 9.
11. Design Action—Action to reduce risk priority number.
12. Design Validation—Method to verify the design motion.

Figure 7-8. This chart shows a step-by-step process for performing failure mode and effects analysis (FMEA). The Joint Commission Resources book titled *Failure Mode and Effects Analysis (FMEA): Proactive Risk Reduction* provides detailed guidance on this proactive approach to risk reduction. See the Selected Bibliography.

Source: Juran JM, Gryna FM: *Juran's Quality Control Handbook*, 4th ed. New York: McGraw-Hill, Inc., 1988. Used with permission.

Tool Profile:
Fault tree analysis
(Synonym: tree diagram)
(See Figure 7-9, below.)

Stage to Use: Identifying proximate causes; identifying root causes; identifying opportunities for improvement.

Purpose: To provide a systematic way of prospectively examining a design or process for possible ways in which failure can occur and provide a graphic display of an event and the event's contributing factors.

Simple Steps to Success:
1. Define the top event of interest.
2. Construct the fault tree for the top event. List the major contributory factors under the top event as the first-level branches.
3. Continue the branching process by adding another level to the tree. These are the factors that might have accounted for the first-level branches.
4. Add additional levels of branching, as necessary.
5. Validate the tree diagram. Review the visualized events for accuracy and completeness.
6. Modify the diagram, as necessary. Retest the modified diagram.
7. Analyze the tree diagram. Identify possible problem scenarios.

Tips for Effective Use
- Generally, the contributory factors can be grouped under such headings as personnel, material or equipment, procedures/processes, and so on.
- To validate the diagram, follow each of the paths through the tree for its "fit" with the facts of the sentinel event or accident. Is each factor plausible?
- Test and retest the tree diagram to "prune" the tree.
- The best-fit scenario will be the scenario most likely to have resulted in the problem in terms of probability and/or the known facts of the particular situation.
- The root cause can be identified based on the inadequacies (causes) identified when listing possible scenarios.
- Corrective or preventive actions should be based on the event and root cause determination.

8. Select the scenario that best fits the facts of the sentinel event or problem.
9. Determine the root cause of the event.
10. Recommend corrective and/or preventive actions.

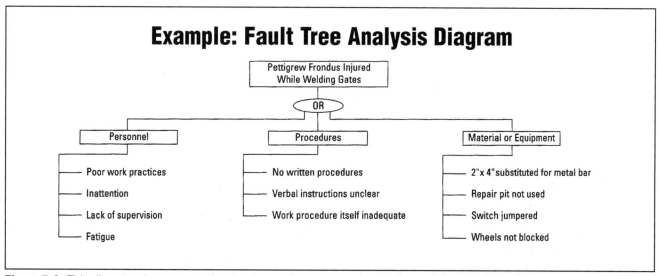

Figure 7-9. This diagram shows a fault tree constructed for a situation in which a maintenance worker was injured while making repairs. The first-level branches are divided into personnel, procedures, and material/equipment categories.
Source: Wilson PF, Dell LD, Anderson GF: *Root Cause Analysis: A Tool for Total Quality Management*. Milwaukee: ASQC Quality Press, 1993, p 179. Used with permission.

Tool Profile:
Flowchart
(See Figure 7-10, page 157.)

Stage to Use: Identifying proximate causes; identifying root causes; identifying opportunities for improvement; implementing and monitoring improvements.

Purpose: To help teams understand all steps in a process through the use of common, easily recognizable symbols; this illustrates the actual path a process takes or the ideal path it should follow.

Simple Steps to Success:

1. Define the process to be charted and establish starting and ending points of the process.
2. Brainstorm activities and decision points in the process. Look for specific activities and decisions necessary to keep the process moving to its conclusion.
3. Determine the sequence of activities and decision points.
4. Use the information to create the flowchart. Place each activity in a box and place each decision point in a diamond. Connect these with lines and arrows to indicate the flow of the process.
5. Analyze the flowchart. Look for unnecessary steps, redundancies, black holes, barriers, and any other difficulties.

Tips for Effective Use

- Ensure that the flowchart is constructed by the individuals actually performing the work being charted.
- Be sure to examine a process within a system, rather than the system itself.
- If the process seems daunting and confusing, create a simple high-level flowchart containing only the most basic components. Do not include too much detail; be wary of obscuring the basic process with too many minor components.
- Use adhesive notes placed on a wall to experiment with sequence until the appropriate one is determined.
- Make the chart the basis for designing an improved process, using spots where the process works well as models for improvement.
- Create a separate flowchart that represents the ideal path of the process, and then compare the two charts for discrepancies.
- Keep in mind that difficulties probably reflect confusion in the process being charted, and work through them.

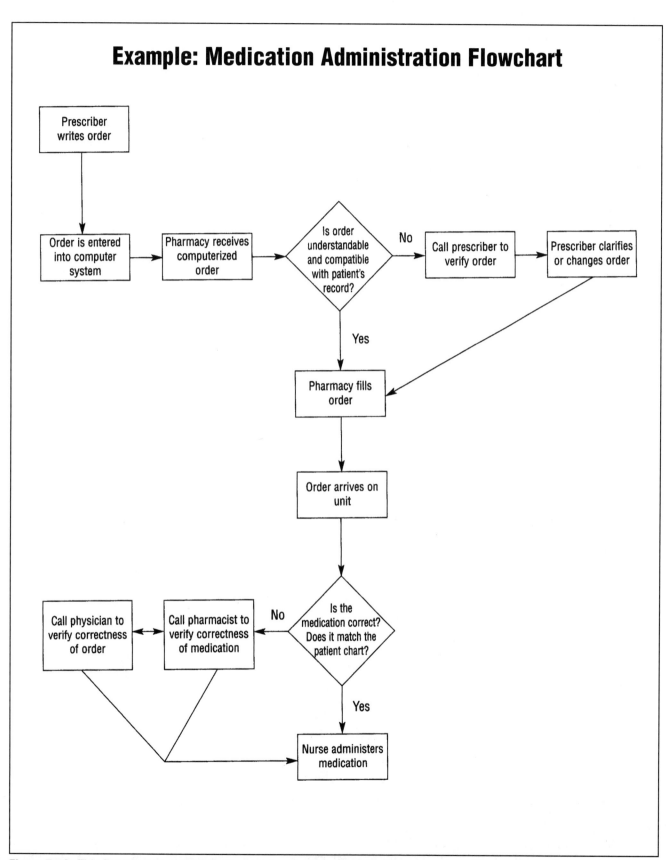

Example: Medication Administration Flowchart

Figure 7-10. This flowchart shows the basic steps in a traditional medication use system. The process components are arranged sequentially, and each stage can be expanded as necessary to show all possible steps.

Tool Profile:
Gantt chart
(See Figure 7-11, below.)

Stage to Use: Identifying proximate causes; identifying root causes; identifying opportunities for improvement; implementing and monitoring improvements.

Purpose: To graphically depict the time line for long-term and complex projects, enabling a team to gauge its progress.

Simple Steps to Success:

1. Agree on start and stop dates for the project, and outline its major steps.
2. Draw a time line.
3. Write the first step of the project under the appropriate time period. Enclose it in a rectangle long enough to stretch across the length of time estimated for completion.
4. Do the same for each of the succeeding steps.

Tips for Effective Use

- Leave enough space in the time line to write beneath each time period.
- Write entries in a stair-step fashion, each step below the one before it, so that overlapping steps are clearly indicated.
- Color in the rectangles as each step is completed.
- If the project is very complex and lengthy, consider creating a Gantt chart for each phase or each quarter of the year.

EXAMPLE: Gantt Chart

Task: Design Phase	Person(s) Responsible	Apr	May	Jun	Jul	Aug	Sep	Oct	Nov	Dec
Identify and appoint credentialing committee	SH	■								
Identify performance measures	SH and SR		■						■	■
Define policies and procedures that outline appointment, reappointment, and privileging process	SH and SR		■	■						
Develop credentialing application	SH and SR			■						

Figure 7-11. This Gantt chart of a competency and privileging process helped one team to determine what tasks to undertake in what order. The chart details the target date and person(s) responsible for each task in the development process.

Tool Profile:
Histogram
(See Figure 7-12, page 160.)

Stage to Use: Identifying proximate causes; identifying root causes; identifying opportunities for improvement; implementing and monitoring improvements.

Purpose: To provide a snapshot of the way data are distributed within a range of values and the amount of variation within a given process, suggesting where to focus improvement efforts.

Simple Steps to Success:
1. Obtain the data sets and count the number of data points.
2. Determine the range for the entire data set.
3. Set the number of classes into which the data will be divided.
4. Determine the class width (by dividing the range by the number of classes).
5. Establish class boundaries.
6. Construct the histogram.
7. Count the data points in each class and create the bars.
8. Analyze the findings.

Tips for Effective Use
- Data should be variable (that is, measured on a continuous scale such as temperature, time, weight, speed, and so forth).
- Make sure data are representative of typical and current conditions.
- Use more than 50 data points to ensure the emergence of meaningful patterns.
- Be sure that the classes are mutually exclusive so that each data point will fit into only one class.
- Using K=10 class intervals makes for easier mental calculations.
- Be aware that the number of intervals can influence the pattern of the sample.
- To construct the histogram, place the values for the classes on the horizontal axis and the frequency on the vertical axis.
- Be suspicious of the accuracy of the data if the histogram suddenly stops at one point without some previous decline in the data.
- Remember that some processes are naturally skewed; do not expect a "normal" pattern every time.
- Large variability or skewed distribution may signal that the process requires further attention.
- Take time to think of alternative explanations for the patterns seen in the histogram.

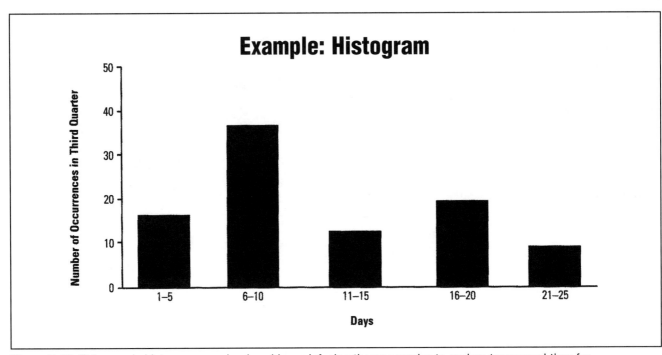

Figure 7-12. This sample histogram was developed by an infusion therapy service to analyze turnaround time for authenticating verbal orders from physicians. The irregular distribution suggests opportunities for improvement.

Tool Profile:
Multivoting
(See Figure 7-13, below.)

Stage to Use: Identifying proximate causes; identifying root causes; identifying opportunities for improvement.

Purpose: To narrow down a broad list of ideas (that is, more than ten) to those that are most important and worthy of immediate attention. This involves reaching a team consensus about a list frequently generated by brainstorming.

Simple Steps to Success:
1. Combine any items on a brainstorming or other list that are the same or similar.
2. Assign letters to items on the new list.
3. Determine the number of points that will be assigned to the list by each group member. Each member will use a predetermined number of points (typically between five and ten) to vote on the

different items on the list.
4. Allow time for group members to assign points independently.
5. Indicate each member's point allocation on the list.
6. Tally the votes.
7. Note items with the greatest number of points.
8. Choose the final group or multivote again.

Tips for Effective Use
- Ensure that when combining ideas on the lists, the team members who suggested the idea agree with the new wording.
- Use letters rather than numbers to identify each statement so that team members do not become confused by the voting process.
- Clearly define each idea so that it is easily understood by everyone voting.

Example: Multivoting

Improvement Opportunities	Number of Votes
A. Facility safety management	3
B. Patient education	7
C. Staff orientation	5
D. Referral (authorization)	3
E. Care coordination and communication	1
F. Laundry	7
G. Medication profile	5

Figure 7-13. This figure shows the results of multivoting on priorities for improvement at an Indian health center. The team was able to reach consensus on the need for prioritizing the laundering process.

Tool Profile:
Pareto chart
(See Figure 7-14, page 163.)

Stage to Use: Identifying root causes; identifying opportunities for improvement.

Purpose: To show which events or causes are most frequent and therefore have the greatest effect. This enables a team to determine what problems to solve and in what order.

Simple Steps to Success:

1. Decide on a topic of study. The topic can be any outcome for which a number of potential causes has been identified.
2. Select causes or conditions to be compared. Identify the factors that contribute to the outcome—the more specific the better.
3. Set the standard for comparison. In many cases, this will be frequency, although factors may be compared based on their cost or quantity.
4. Collect data. Determine how often each factor occurs (or the cost or quantity of each, as appropriate). Use a check sheet to help with this task.
5. Make the comparison. Based on the data collected in the previous step, compare the factors and rank them from most to least.
6. Draw the chart's vertical axis. On the left side of the chart, draw a vertical line and mark the standard of measurement in increments.
7. List factors along the horizontal axis. Factors should be arranged in descending order, with the highest ranking factor at the far left.
8. Draw a bar for each factor. The bars represent how often each factor occurs, the cost of each factor, or its quantity, as applicable.
9. Include additional features, if desired. By making a few simple additions to the chart, a team can show the cumulative frequency, cost, or quantity of the categories in percentages.

Tips for Effective Use

- If the team is working from a cause-and-effect diagram, the topic will be the effect that has been targeted for improvement.
- When selecting factors for comparison, beware of grouping several distinct problems together, which can skew the rank order. Refer to the cause-and-effect diagram, and use the most specific causes and factors possible.
- Be sure to mark the chart clearly to show the standard of measurement.
- When analyzing the chart, keep in mind that numbers do not always tell the whole story. Sometimes 2 severe complaints deserve more attention than 100 minor complaints.

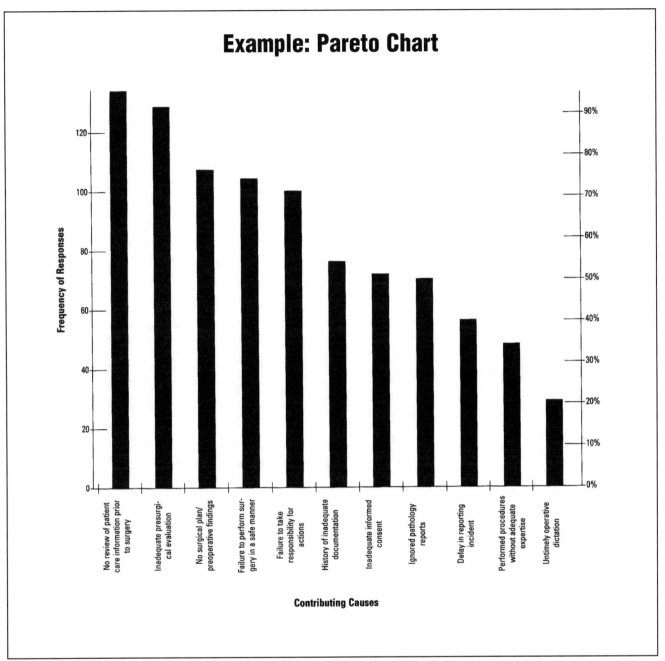

Example: Pareto Chart

Figure 7-14. One organization used a Pareto chart to rank the frequency of responses of selected root causes provided by team members investigating a sentinel event involving a wrong-site surgery.

Used with permission.

Tool Profile:
Run chart
(See Figure 7-15, below.)

Stage to Use: Identifying proximate causes; identifying root causes; implementing and monitoring improvements.

Purpose: To identify trends and patterns in a process over a specific period of time so that teams can identify areas that require or are experiencing improvement.

Simple Steps to Success:
1. Decide what the chart will measure (what data will be collected over what period of time).
2. Draw the graph's axes.
3. Plot the data points and connect them with a line.
4. Plot the center line (that is, the overall average of all measurements).
5. Evaluate the chart to identify meaningful trends.
6. Investigate the findings.

Tips for Effective Use
- Make sure that the time period for data display is long enough to show a trend.
- Use at least enough data points to ensure detection of meaningful patterns or trends.
- Clearly mark all units of measurement on the chart. The x axis should indicate time or sequence; the y axis should indicate what is being studied.
- Indicate significant changes or events by drawing dashed lines through the chart at the appropriate points on the x axis.
- Do not be too concerned with any one particular point on the chart (that is, wild points); instead, focus on vital changes in the process.
- Be aware that a "run" of six or more points on one side of the average indicates an important event or change.
- Integrate favorable changes into the system; take action to improve performance of unfavorable changes.

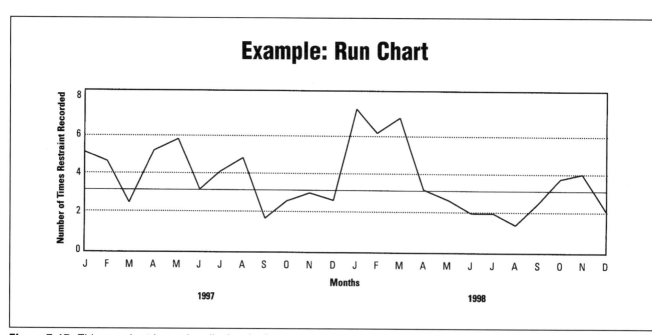

Figure 7-15. This run chart is used to display the frequency of restraint use for psychiatric patients.

Tool Profile:

Scatter diagram
(Synonym: scattergram)
(See Figure 7-16, page 166.)

Stage to Use: Identifying root causes; implementing and monitoring improvements.

Purpose: To display the correlation—not necessarily the cause-and-effect relationship—between two variables.

Simple Steps to Success:

1. Decide which two variables will be tested.
2. Collect and record relevant data. Gather 50 to 100 paired samples of data involving each of the variables, and record them on a data sheet.
3. Draw the horizontal and vertical axes.
4. Plot the variables on the graph. If a value is repeated, circle that point as many times as necessary.
5. Interpret the completed diagram.

Tips for Effective Use

- Select two variables with a suspected relationship (for example, delays in processing tests and total volume of tests to be processed).
- Use the horizontal (x) axis for the variable you suspect is the cause and the vertical (y) axis for the effect.
- Construct the graph so that values increase while moving up and to the right of each axis.
- The more the clusters form a straight line (which could be diagonal), the stronger the relationship between the two variables.
- If points cluster in an area running from lower left to upper right, the two variables have a positive correlation. This means that an increase in y may depend on an increase in x; if you can control x, you have a good chance of controlling y.
- If points cluster from upper left to lower right, the variables have a negative correlation. This means that as x increases y may decrease.
- If points are scattered all over the diagram, these variables may not have any correlation (the effect, y, may be dependent on a variable other than x).
- Remember, if the diagram indicates a relationship, it is not necessarily a cause-and-effect relationship.
- Be aware that even if the data do not appear to have a relationship, they may be related.
- Although scatter diagrams can not prove a causal relationship between two variables, they can offer persuasive evidence.

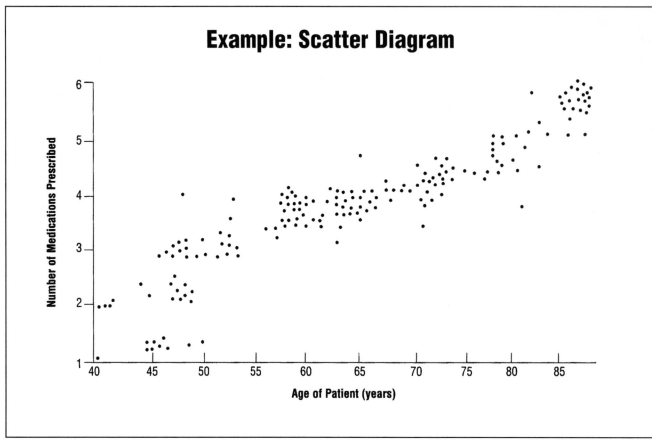

Figure 7-16. This scatter diagram compares two variables associated with self-administration errors—the number of medications prescribed and the ages of the patients involved. As might be expected, the clustering of points shows that the older the patient, the higher the number of medications involved in care.

Tool Profile:
Time line
(See Figure 7-17, below.)

Stage to Use: Identifying proximate causes; identifying root causes.

Purpose: To graphically display the temporal sequence of events.

Simple Steps to Success:
1. Draw a horizontal line across a piece of paper.
2. Establish time increments and note these on the horizontal line as vertical hatch marks.
3. Using arrows or vertical lines, note the major events at the appropriate point along the time line.
4. Using arrows or vertical lines, note the major actions at the appropriate point along the time line.

Tips for Effective Use
- Ask each key witness of an event to create a separate time line. Compare these for patterns of agreement and disagreement.
- Separation of actions and events enhances the legibility of the time line.
- You may wish to create a time line of the ideal sequence of events and actions and then, in order to identify risk points and problems, compare this to the time line of actual events and actions.

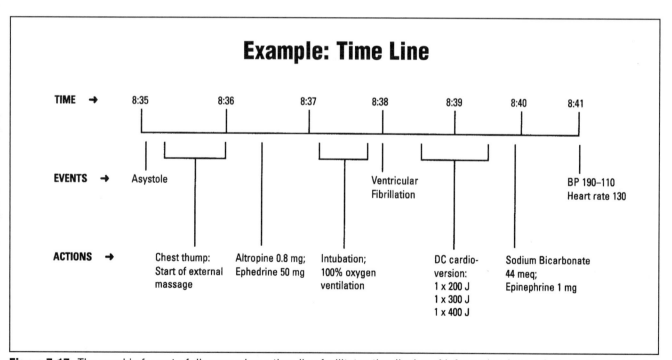

Figure 7-17. The graphic format of diagramming a time line facilitates the display of information from a fast-moving incident. Readability is enhanced by the separation of actions and events. In this example, the time, events, and actions taken to handle an intraoperative cardiac arrest are displayed.

Source: Caplan RA: In-depth analysis of anesthetic mishaps: Tools and techniques. *Int Anesthesiol Clin* 27(3):157, 1989.

Chapter 8

Case Study: A Sample Infant Abduction Root Cause Analysis

Case at a Glance

Organization:

St. Joseph's Hospital and Medical Center*
Paterson, New Jersey

Type and Size of Facility:

Acute care hospital with approximately 800 beds, a
level 2 trauma center, a level 3 regional perinatal
center, and a 30-bed combined postpartum/newborn
nursery unit.

Staff and Services:

Hospital has approximately 4,100 full- and part-time
employees and averages approximately 26,000
admissions per year; postpartum/newborn nursery unit
has a cross-trained staff of 70 and averages
approximately 2,700 deliveries per year.

Sentinel Event:

Infant abduction from the postpartum unit.

Framework for Investigation:

Root cause analysis performed by a total quality
management team using Juran's six-step improvement
process. (See Sidebar 8-1 right, for the key steps St.
Joseph's team used in its root cause analysis and
improvement actions.)

Common-Cause Issues:

Security process/system
Patient and staff education

---

* Editor's note: Our sincere thanks to the staff at St. Joseph's Hospital and
  Medical Center in Paterson, New Jersey. Their goal here is to share their
  experience to assist colleagues at other organizations.

Sidebar 8-1. Key Steps in St. Joseph's Root Cause Analysis and Improvement Strategy

- Implement Infant Abduction Policy.
- Secure leadership involvement and support.
- Define the sentinel event problem.
- Define the team's risk reduction mission.
- Form a team to investigate the event.
- Address team's improvement focus, staff concerns, and confidentiality.
- Identify framework for investigation.
- Establish schedule and activities for root cause analysis.
- Conduct and review literature search.
- Identify proximate causes.
- Create flowcharts of critical processes, identifying risk points and possible root causes.
- Brainstorm about risk points and create cause-and-effect diagrams of root cause theories.
- Establish and implement a data collection plan.
- Collect and analyze data.
- Formulate root causes based on data analysis.
- Identify improvement strategies using a literature search, benchmark study, data and flowchart analysis, and other means.
- Define improvement criteria.
- Identify improvements most likely to be effective.
- Recommend specific improvements to hospital leadership.
- Develop an improvement implementation plan.
- Implement improvement plan.
- Monitor improvement plan.

Tools and Techniques Used:
Bar graph, brainstorming, benchmarking, cause-and-effect diagram, control chart, failure mode and effects analysis, flowchart, literature surveillance, prioritization matrix, tree diagram

The Event

On the morning of August 20, 1997, a female visitor, using a visitor's pass, entered the postpartum/newborn nursery unit of St. Joseph's Hospital and Medical Center in Paterson, New Jersey. To obtain the pass, she had provided an actual patient's name and room number. The visitor entered a new mother's room. The mother had been discharged and was awaiting transportation home. The visitor befriended the mother and spent a couple of hours in the room talking with the mother.

Initial Response

At approximately noon, the visitor suggested to the mother that the mother use the bathroom, perhaps to take a shower or to smoke. The visitor told the mother that she would watch the baby. The mother used the bathroom. When she emerged an unspecified amount of time later, the visitor and baby were not in the room. The mother went to the nursery and asked the staff for her baby.

When the staff could not locate the baby, they enacted the hospital's Infant Abduction Policy. This policy addresses communication and security issues following an abduction. It provides a clear protocol on how the event should be reported: The nurse manager covering the unit reports the event to the director who notifies the vice president for patient care services, and on up the chain of command. It also specifies that the investigation is handled by the security department, working with the local police department.

Immediately following notification, communication and investigation commenced according to hospital policy. Staff moved the mother to another unit, and visitors were kept to a minimum. Police, having been informed

according to hospital policy, arrived on the scene to gather evidence and question staff. Due to the criminal nature of the event, preservation of evidence was handled by the police department in coordination with the security department.

The outcome? A member of the abductor's family, having seen coverage of the event on television and observing the family member with an unfamiliar newborn infant, informed the local police. Authorities returned the baby to the mother in safe condition by 10:30 PM that same day. The baby was still wearing the hospital's identification band. Videotapes from the surveillance cameras in the hospital's lobby, reviewed by the police, were helpful in identifying the abductor, who also had visited the hospital the day prior to the abduction.

Determining What Happened and Why

Immediately following the event, the director of maternal-child nursing, the director of quality management, the vice president for patient care services, and the unit's nurse manager started brainstorming about possible members of a root cause analysis team. They decided to use a total quality management (TQM) team approach with cross-hierarchical, cross-functional representation from staff involved in baby handling and safety.

Individuals selected for the team were the director of maternal-child nursing (who served as the leader), the director of quality management (who served as the facilitator), the nurse manager of a sister unit, two staff nurses on duty during the abduction, the unit's receptionist, a nurse's aide, the director of security, a security guard, the on-site supervisor of the agency providing the hospital's security guard staff, an information desk staff member, and the supervisor of the information desk.

The first team meeting was highly emotional, with everyone shaken by the event. Time was spent reassuring team members that the hospital was seriously interested in looking at the systems and processes related to the protection of infants and in identifying ways to improve them. The vice president of patient care services attended the first meeting to set the tone and reassure the team that the senior administration was not seeking to lay blame or to look for scapegoats but that improvement would be the focus; these extensive efforts were both critical and successful. The team also discussed use of Juran's six-step process and ground rules, including the need for strict confidentiality throughout the root cause analysis process.

Working within the Joint Commission's then-30 day requirement for completion of a root cause analysis,* the team established an aggressive schedule with two- to three-hour meetings three times a week and additional behind-the-scenes work. For example, after the team agreed to get a literature search under way during an early meeting, the postpartum nurse manager, a team member, directed the search, reviewed the relevant articles, and distributed them to team members before the team's next meeting. Similarly, after the team agreed on a particular data collection effort, a team member established the data collection plan, collected the data, entered them in the computer, analyzed them, and presented the data in graphic format by the following week. Attendance was not a problem; when necessary, the staff's schedules were modified so that team members could participate to the fullest extent.

Prior to the sentinel event, there were measures in place to assure proper identification of visitors. When a visitor entered the hospital, he or she stopped at the information desk in the main lobby for a visitor's pass, and proceeded upstairs one floor to the postpartum newborn nursery unit. Upon entering the unit, the visitor would walk past the postpartum nursing station, staffed by a unit receptionist, and to his or her destination. The

unit is not now and was not then locked, and mothers can room in with the baby 24 hours a day. Visiting hours are flexible, and the unit is relatively open in terms of access for both staff and hospital visitors.

During an initial meeting, the team defined the sentinel event problem as follows: "A discharged mother gave her newborn baby to an unauthorized person, who left St. Joseph's Hospital and Medical Center with the baby." The team's mission was to significantly reduce the risk of another infant abduction by conducting a thorough and credible root cause analysis and implementing meaningful improvement strategies.

The team identified two proximate causes contributing to the risk of baby abduction: unauthorized persons on the postpartum unit, who may or may not have a pass, and babies in the care of the mother, who leave them unattended. "Unattended" was defined as a baby in a room with no authorized person present or the mother present, but asleep. When the first situation coexists with the second, the situation is volatile.

The team began by creating flowcharts for three identified critical processes:
- Control of babies born in the hospital from the moment of birth to their discharge;
- Control of babies born outside of the hospital from transport to discharge; and
- Control of visitors at all times (see Figure 8-1, page 172).

The team reviewed and analyzed the charts for what they called "brick walls" and "black holes"—the risk points or obstacles in the processes. Two issues emerged:
- There were ways for individuals to subvert the visitor security process to gain access to the postpartum unit. Individuals could obtain visitor passes under false pretenses.
- Despite adequate and repeated reminders from the staff, mothers left their rooming-in babies unattended.

---

* The current Joint Commission requirement for submission of a thorough and credible root cause analysis is 45 days. The root cause analysis includes an action plan. The actions itemized in this plan are both those completed within the 45 days and those planned for the future. All actions need not be completed within the 45-day period. Visit the Joint Commission's Web site at www.jcaho.org for the most up-to-date information on the Sentinel Event Policy.

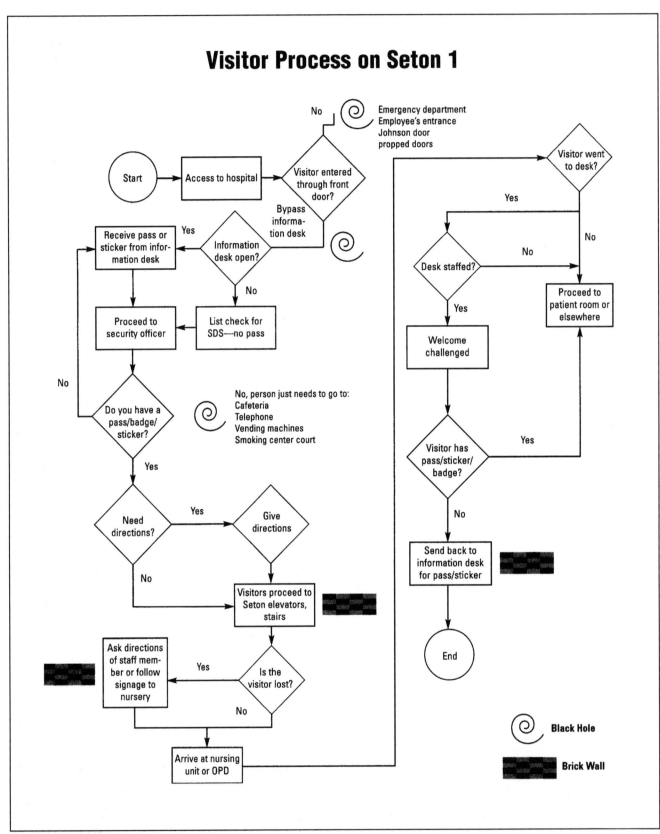

Figure 8-1. This flowchart shows the visitor flow during and after hours. Note the symbols used to identify risk points and obstacles in the process, called "black holes" and "brick walls."

Source: St. Joseph's Hospital and Medical Center, Paterson, NJ. Used with permission.

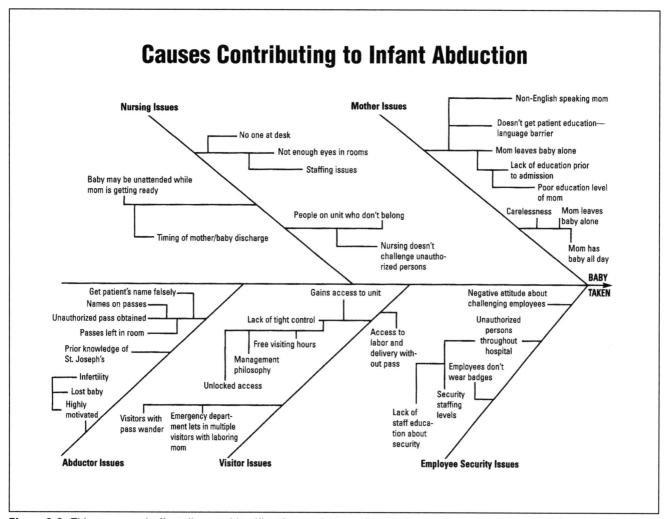

Causes Contributing to Infant Abduction

Figure 8-2. This cause-and-effect diagram identifies the nursing, mother, visitor, employee security, and abductor issues involved in an abduction of a baby from the hospital.

Source: St. Joseph's Hospital and Medical Center, Paterson, NJ. Used with permission.

To pursue these issues further and to begin to answer the questions "How can unauthorized persons access the unit?" and "Why are babies left unattended?" the team conducted a brainstorming session in which a number of theories were developed. The team then constructed a cause-and-effect diagram based on its theories (see Figure 8-2 above).

To test the theories, the team organized a six-day data collection effort aimed at determining the incidence of unauthorized visitors on the unit and the incidence of unattended babies. Two studies—a security study and a nursing study—were conducted. The data collection tool used by the security staff appears as Figure 8-3,

page 174. The tool used by the nursing assistant appears as Figure 8-4, page 175.

The findings surprised the team. Despite the high level of emotion and publicity surrounding the event in the weeks following the abduction, data indicated that unauthorized persons could have access to the unit and some babies were still left unattended by their mothers. The team was surprised that babies were found unattended even after the education provided to the staff and enhanced surveillance efforts. Within the study period, there were 4 instances out of 168 observations of babies left unattended; the mothers were either asleep or in the bathroom. When the

Security Data Collection Tool

	Individuals With Pass	Individuals Without Pass			No ID Badge		
		Sent Back	Lost	Outpatient	Resident	MD	Employee
1200–0100							
0100–0200							
0200–0300							
0300–0400							
0400–0500							
0500–0600							
0600–0700							
0700–0800							
0800–0900							
0900–1000							
1000–1100							
1100–1200							
1200–1300							
1300–1400							
1400–1500							
1500–1600							
1600–1700							
1700–1800							
1800–1900							
1900–2000							
2000–2100							
2100–2200							
2200–2300							
2300–0000							

Figure 8-3. This data collection tool was used in the security study to record the incidence of unauthorized visitors on the labor and delivery unit, among other information.

Source: St. Joseph's Hospital and Medical Center, Paterson, NJ. Used with permission.

nursing assistant collecting the data discovered an unattended baby, the assistant stayed with the baby until the mother woke or emerged, talked with the mother, and reemphasized the importance of never leaving the baby unattended. The team concluded that unauthorized persons on the unit and unattended babies were root causes of potential abductions. A bar graph used to display data collected in the security study appears as Figure 8-5, page 176. A summary of both the security and nursing studies appears as Figure 8-6, page 177.

Designing and Implementing Improvement Strategies

The team moved quickly to identify possible improvement strategies or "remedies." A literature search effort was key at this stage. Through the hospital's Health Sciences Library and a nonprofit research organization in Washington, D.C., the team obtained 12 articles from the professional literature on infant abduction listed in Sidebar 8-2, page 178. The literature demonstrated that it was not uncommon for abductors to find a way to bypass the

Nursing Data Collection Tool

Baby Safety Team
Study Period: 07:01 AM Tuesday 9/2/97 to 07:00 AM Tuesday 9/9/97

Instructions: A nursing assistant is assigned on every shift to collect data for their entire shift during the study period. During breaks, the data collection needs to be assigned to a covering nursing assistant. One time during each hour of the shift, the assigned nursing assistant will make rounds in every room on the unit and record the number of babies in each category.

Time/Date: _____	Number of babies rooming in on the unit	Number of babies with mom or dad in attendance	Number of babies unattended (if mother is asleep, count baby as unattended)	Number of babies with only roommate (if roommate is sleeping, count baby as unattended)	Number of babies with visitor in attendance (with pass)
07:01–08:00					
08:01–09:00					
09:01–10:00					
10:01–11:00					
11:01–12:00					
12:01–13:00					
13:01–14:00					
14:01–15:00					
Data collector day shift:					
15:01–16:00					
16:01–17:00					
17:01–18:00					
18:01–19:00					
19:01–20:00					
20:01–21:00					
21:01–22:00					
22:01–23:00					
Data collector evening shift:					
23:01–00:00					
00:01–01:00					
01:01–02:00					
02:01–03:00					
03:01–04:00					
04:01–05:00					
05:01–06:00					
06:01–07:00					
Data collector night shift:					

Figure 8-4. This data collection tool was used by nursing assistants to record the number of babies rooming in at any given hour and the number of those babies left unattended.

Source: St. Joseph's Hospital and Medical Center, Paterson, NJ. Used with permission.

security system and befriend the patient. The team identified an inventory of remedies described in the literature.

One article described a simple card-receipt system used in a hospital in Arkansas for infant security, which involves retaining a card in the nursery for each baby

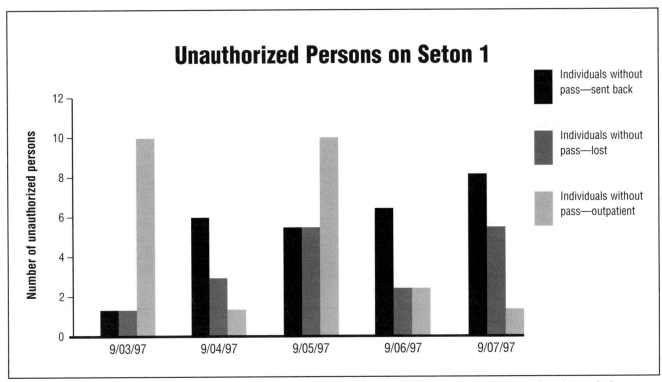

Figure 8-5. This bar graph displays the number of unauthorized persons in the postpartum unit over a five-day period.
Source: St. Joseph's Hospital and Medical Center, Paterson, NJ. Used with permission.

rooming in with a mother.[1] The team reviewed the system and, due to its low cost and easy setup, implemented the new system immediately. While the steps of the Juran TQM process were followed in detail, corrective/preventive actions were taken throughout. The team also conducted a benchmarking study to identify remedies used by neighboring hospitals. The director of maternal-child nursing called 14 hospitals to explore the systems they used for infant security. She asked about their use of technological security systems and learned about what they liked and did not like about the systems. They all either already had a technological baby security system or were evaluating systems with the intention of purchasing one. All hospitals with the technological systems in place acknowledged their ease of use and effectiveness; criticisms of the various systems were minimal.

The team supplemented the list of potential remedies identified through benchmarking and the literature search by analyzing the process flowcharts and data collected from the studies. The team used failure mode and effects analysis and a prioritization matrix to select the improvements likely to be the most effective (see Figures 8-7 and 8-8, pages 179 and 180).

Criteria used to select improvements based on these and other analyses included the option's consistency with the hospital's mission and values, ability to bolster the present security systems without presenting an environment that might be viewed by patients and families as a "locked fortress," possibility of failure, ability to bolster present educational efforts, ability to reduce risks, and cost to implement. The team recommended to the hospital's quality council 15 specific improvements, focusing on security process or system changes and educational efforts. In the area of security process and system changes, the team recommended the following:

- Removing names from visitor identification passes, leaving only room numbers to help reduce the likelihood of individuals getting unauthorized passes.

Analysis of Data Collection Efforts

Baby Safety Team

Data Collection 9/2/97 to 9/7/97

Analyses of the process flowcharts and cause-and-effect diagrams pointed to two primary areas of concern: unauthorized visitors on Seton 1 [labor and delivery unit] and unattended babies. Although worrisome in and of themselves, the combination of unauthorized visitors and unattended babies provides opportunity for baby abduction. Security and nursing studies were conducted to analyze the present potential.

Security Study

Security guards in plain clothes, with an ID as patient representatives,* were posted at the entrance of Seton 1 and collected data for a six-day period of time. Data from the first day did not represent the entire 24 hours, and was consequently not used in this analysis. The guards recorded the incidence of visitors on the unit properly identified with passes, unauthorized persons attempting to access the unit without a pass (and the nature of their business, that is, lost, sent back, or outpatient), and staff members who were not identified with an ID (resident, physician, or employee).

The plainclothes security officer who collected the data advised all unidentified staff members of the need to go to the security department for a temporary ID during the data collection period.

Key findings from the security study include the following:
- Visitor activity fluctuates from 75 to 150 persons during any given 24-hour period.
- Visitors with legitimate passes were allowed access to the unit. However, the study did not determine if any visitor accessed a pass in some false manner.
- As few as 1 and as many as 14 staff members without IDs were present on Seton 1 during the five days of the study. The incidence was greatest among physicians making rounds on Sunday.
- Unauthorized persons attempting to access Seton 1 were made up of those outpatients who were lost, other persons without passes who were "lost," and those without passes who were sent back.
- The number of outpatients fluctuated with the day of the week; weekend days had fewer lost outpatients than weekdays.

- Individuals without passes (sent back or lost) varied from 0 to 10 in any given 24-hour period.

It is clear that the 24-hour security guard presence assisted greatly in reducing the potential for unauthorized persons on Seton 1. However, the volume of visitors presents a potential risk factor. In addition, the security guard cannot guarantee that every individual with a pass is a truly legitimate visitor.

Nursing Study

Nursing assistants were assigned to conduct an hourly assessment 24 hours a day, 6 days a week. Nursing assistants were to record the number of babies who were "rooming in" at any given hour and the number of babies left unattended by the mother (that is, the mother went to the bathroom, used the shower, or fell asleep). Assistants were to record those incidents when the baby was left under the observation of the roommate or a visitor.

In the course of data collection, if any unattended babies in the care of the mother were uncovered, nursing assistants were instructed to stay with the baby until the mother returned and re-instruct the mother in safety precautions using good guest relations skills.

Because analyses of the cause-and-effect diagram and the process flowcharts did not turn up any potential risk factors in the nursery security system (that is, locks on nursery doors, nurse presence with infants at all times, no babies ever unattended in the nursery), the nursing study was restricted to rooming-in babies in the care of their mothers.

Key findings from the nursing study include the following:
- Of the 168 observation periods, there were 4 instances when babies (rooming in, in the care of their mothers) were found to be unattended;
- The number of babies "rooming in" at any given time ranged from 7 to 17; and
- There were no incidences of babies left unattended by the roommate or by a visitor.

The study demonstrates that, although rare, there are instances when babies (rooming in, in the care of their mothers) are unattended.

---

* The security officer was posted in this manner so as not to instill a sense of fear in patients.

Figure 8-6. This summary report includes a description of security and nursing data collection studies, key findings, and analysis of the data.

Source: St. Joseph's Hospital and Medical Center, Paterson, NJ. Used with permission.

<table>
<tr><td>

Sidebar 8-2. St. Joseph's Infant Abduction Literature Search

The following articles were used by staff of St. Joseph's in conducting a root cause analysis and developing an action plan in response to an infant abduction.

Bainbridge M: Another way to keep postpartum and nursery units safe. *RN* 54:9–10, Sep 1991.

Beachy P, Deacon J: Preventing neonatal kidnapping. *J Obstet Gynecol Neonatal Nurs* 21:12–16, Jan-Feb 1992.

Davis P: Other precautions to protect newborns. *RN* 55:13, Mar 1992.

Dextradeur CC, Godfrey TM: A badge of security. *MCN Am J Matern Child Nurs* 16:175–176, May-Jun 1991.

Eubanks P: Hospital nursery kidnappings are rare but devastating. *Hospitals* 64:64, 66, Jun 20, 1990.

Goodwin TC, Simmons J: Our simple system keeps newborns safe. *RN* 54:17–18, 20, May 1991.

Myrabo J: Neonatal kidnapping. *J Obstet Gyneonatal Nurs* 22:105, Mar-Apr 1993.

Pallarito K: More hospitals drop practice of sending birth announcements. *Modern Healthcare* 22:38, Apr 13, 1992.

Rabun JB: Preventing neonatal kidnapping. *J Obstet Gyneonatal Nurs* 22:15–16, Jan-Feb 1993.

Shuman M: Kidnapped kids a possible nightmare. *Modern Healthcare* 24:28, Feb 21, 1994.

Stephenson T: Abduction of infants from hospitals: Vigilance and staff training are the keys to prevention. *Br Med J* 310:754–755, Mar 25, 1995.

Stevens E: Preventing neonatal kidnapping. *J Obstet Gyneonatal Nurs* 21:350, Sep-Oct 1992.
</td></tr>
</table>

- Keeping the doors to the postpartum unit closed and installing a sensor system that provides an audible signal when someone passes through the doorway.
- Immediately sending a legitimate employee reporting for work without his or her badge to security for a temporary badge.
- Instituting a 24-hour a day, 7-day a week position at the postpartum unit desk for visitor control. Supplied with a patient census updated every 4 hours, a nurse's aide was given the responsibility of checking the identification of every person that entered the unit. This was kept in place for approximately 6 months, until the infant technological system was fully installed, working smoothly, and until staff members were adequately briefed in routinely checking identification (ID) badges and visitors' passes.
- Increasing security patrols: Guards performed an hourly walk-through and challenged staff or visitors not properly identified.
- Developing and implementing a card-receipt system similar to the one described in the literature.
- Revising the hospital's nursery security policy/procedure to include that every mother must state her name, produce a bracelet, and show identification whenever she claims her baby from the nursery.
- Using a four-ID-band baby identification system, which includes two for the baby, one for the mother, and one for the father or significant other, as identified by the mother.
- Purchasing and implementing a technological baby security system, which involves an unobtrusive sensor attached to the baby's umbilical cord that sounds an alarm, causes doors to lock, and elevator doors to lock open if an unauthorized attempt is made to take the baby off the unit.

Regarding staff and patient educational improvements, the team recommended comprehensive ongoing education, which included the following:

- An educational "blitz" with all employees to address their role in controlling unauthorized persons on the unit. The education focused on three key actions:

Failure Mode and Effects Analysis

Product: Obstetrical Care
Feature: Baby Safety

1	2	3	4	5	6	7	8	9
Mode of Failure	**Cause of Failure**	**Effect of Failure**	**Frequency of Failure**	**Degree of Severity**	**Chance of Detection**	**Risk Priority (4 x 5 x 6 = 7)**	**Design Action**	**Design Validation**
Unauthorized persons	False pass	Get on unit with a pass	1	8	10	80	See Prioritization Matrix	
Unauthorized persons	Wrong door or propped door	Get on unit without a pass	6	6	3	108	See Prioritization Matrix	
Unauthorized persons	Here for one thing, go somewhere else	Get on unit with a sticker or pass	8	6	10	480	See Prioritization Matrix	
Unauthorized persons	Unstaffed desk/staffing	Get on unit with or without pass	2	8	8	128	See Prioritization Matrix	
Unattended baby	Mom in bathroom, shower, falls asleep	Baby available to be taken	1	9	2	18	See Prioritization Matrix	
Unattended baby	Education level low; trust is high	Baby available to be taken	1	10	10	100	See Prioritization Matrix	
Unattended baby	Non-English speaking patients; don't understand the instructions	Baby available to be taken	3	10	10	300	See Prioritization Matrix	

Figure 8-7. The team developed a failure mode and effects analysis and used it in conjunction with a prioritization matrix (Figure 8-8, page 180) to select priorities for improvements. Guidelines for creating a failure mode and effects analysis can be found in Chapter 7, page 153.

Source: St. Joseph's Hospital and Medical Center, Paterson, NJ. Used with permission.

- ○ wearing identification badges at all times,
- ○ questioning those without an ID badge or visitor's pass, and
- ○ preventing unauthorized persons from entering through employee doors;
- • Educating staff through initial and ongoing in-service sessions about the importance of checking the crib card against identification every time a baby is returned to a crib and having the mother state her full name and ID band number when the baby is brought to her;
- • Educating the staff about security issues on an annual basis through an eight-hour seminar titled "Safeguarding Their Tomorrows;" and
- • Enhancing education provided to patients regarding the danger of leaving their babies unattended.

After approval by the quality council, the team developed a full implementation plan, including a time

Prioritization Matrix

	Cost $ = least costly $$$$ = most costly no ranking = no direct cost	Reduce Risk 1 = least possibility of failure 5 = most chance of failure
The technological baby security system involves an infrared sensor attached to the baby's umbilical cord that sounds an alarm, and causes doors to lock and elevator doors to lock open if an attempt is made to leave the unit. Staff must assure that the sensor is not removed as part of the baby discharge process until the mother is literally leaving. This measure would prevent unauthorized persons from leaving with the baby. (In the case of the sentinel event, the baby was discharged and in the mother's care when it was taken.)	$$$	2
Put combination locks or card swipe locks at chapel, coffee shop, and gift shop—alternate entrances that bypass the security officer. (This is one of the brick walls identified in the flow of the visitor process, Figure 8-1.)	$$	3
Remove names from visitor IDs; leave only room numbers. (This is a cause of people getting unauthorized passes listed on the cause-and-effect diagram, Figure 8-2.)		4
Closely monitor doors that are known to be propped (for example, near the mail room, imaging unit.)		5
Conduct an educational/promotional blitz with employees as to their role in controlling unauthorized persons. Their roles are to (1) wear ID badge at all times, (2) question those without ID, (3) do not allow unauthorized persons to enter employee entrances, and (4) do not prop doors open.		4
Go to a four-ID baby identification system, which includes a fourth matching ID band on the father (two on baby, one on mother). This would provide immediate ID to information desk staff and nursing staff.		4
Retrain staff with an in-service on checking the crib card with the ID every time the baby is returned to the crib.		3
Retrain staff with an in-service on having the mother state her full name and ID number when the baby is brought to her.		3
Revise policy/procedure to include patient education regarding caution not to leave baby unattended.		3
Revise policy/procedure to include the need to cite the ID number, produce the bracelet, and show identification when claiming the baby from the nursery.		3
Increase staff to Seton 1 to ensure desk coverage.	$$$$	3
Permanently post a security officer at the Seton 1 entryway 24 hours a day, 7 days per week.	$$$$	4
Validate passes for every visitor on Seton 1 (would need to add staff).	$$$$	5
Lock magnetic doors to Seton 1 at all times. Staff use card swipe; visitors are buzzed in and out.	$$$	3
Monitor and tape all entrances with central monitor in security (similar to the DR).	$$	4
Perform DNA testing for every baby.	$$$	5
Keep fire doors closed at all times (from LDR to Seton 1); staff can hear distinctive "click" when doors are opened.		3
Keep fire doors closed at all times and install automatic door opener with button for stretchers.	$$	3
Increase security patrols on Seton 1.		3
Retrain staff by holding the FBI all-day seminar on infant abduction, "Safeguarding Their Tomorrows," sponsored by Mead Johnson.		3
Establish an identifying card-receipt system (from the literature).		3
Change policy to include, in the event of an abduction, that all phone calls to nursing unit are "diligently screened" at the switchboard (from the literature).		5
Photograph all babies at birth as part of the infant security system. In the event of an abduction, the image can be transmitted to the National Center for Missing and Exploited Children when they distribute the image appropriately. A photography vendor will provide the service free of charge (from the literature and researched with the vendor).		5

Figure 8-8. The Baby Safety Team developed a prioritization matrix to analyze improvement opportunities.

Source: St. Joseph's Hospital and Medical Center, Paterson, NJ. Used with permission.

Tree Diagram

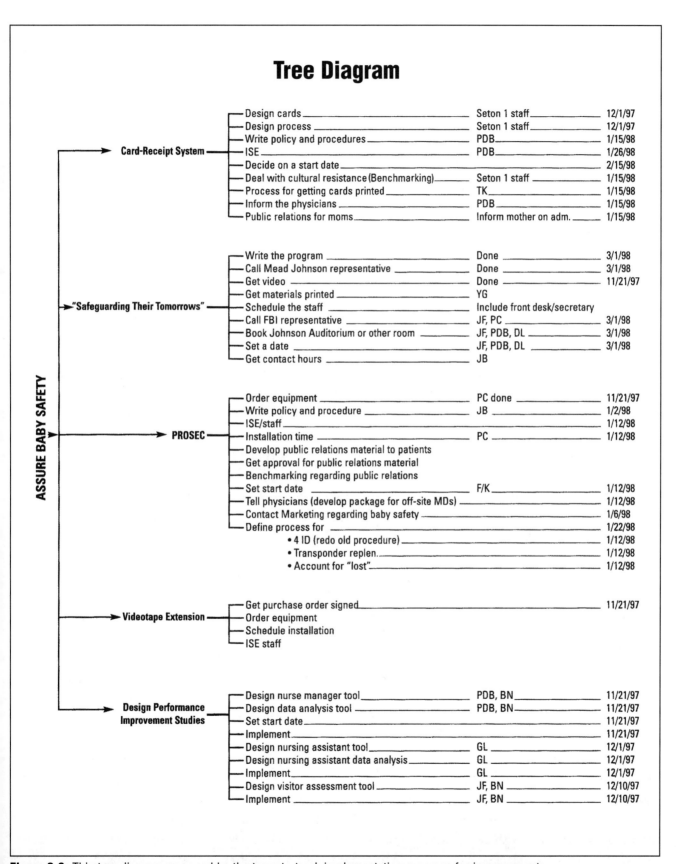

Figure 8-9. This tree diagram was used by the team to track implementation progress for improvements.

Source: St. Joseph's Hospital and Medical Center, Paterson, NJ. Used with permission.

line, and implemented all of the recommended improvements within five months of the infant abduction. The tree diagram used by the team to track implementation progress appears as Figure 8-9, page 181.

Holding the Gains

The team identified seven indicators that would be the focus of continued measurement to track the hospital's success in reducing unauthorized visitors and unattended babies through educational and security process initiatives. Measures included

- whether the mother had been cautioned during her stay not to give her baby to anyone without a proper ID badge with a pink background (a measure of the effectiveness of patient education);
- whether the mother had been cautioned during her stay not to leave her baby unattended (a measure of the effectiveness of patient education);
- whether nursing staff members asked the mother to state her full name when bringing the baby to her (a measure of the effectiveness of staff education);
- whether nursing staff members asked the mother to read the number from her ID band when bringing the baby to her (a measure of the effectiveness of staff education);
- the number of unattended rooming-in babies (a measure of the combined effectiveness of staff and patient education);
- the number of unauthorized persons per hour seeking access to the unit at the postpartum desk (a measure of the effectiveness of the security process improvement); and
- the number of unauthorized persons in patient rooms (a measure of the combined effectiveness of staff education and security process improvements).

Data were collected and analyzed on a weekly basis. The tool used by nurse managers to capture control chart data appears as Figure 8-10, page 183. Data were tracked in control chart format and evaluated by the team and discussed both with the team and the entire postpartum staff. Data collection was performed through three processes involving rounds and a desk assessment:

1. A nurse manager conducted rounds three times per week with a random sampling of 15 mothers/babies on each shift for a total of 45 observations. She asked the mother whether or not nursing staff members asked her to state her full name when bringing the baby to her and whether or not nursing staff members asked her to read the ID number from her ID band when bringing the baby to her. The nurse manager also conducted rounds to 15 randomly selected mothers during the course of the week to ask whether the mothers had been cautioned during their stay not to leave their babies unattended, and whether the mothers had been cautioned during their stay not to give their babies to anyone without a proper ID badge.

2. A nursing assistant conducted walking rounds every hour once a week on all three shifts. She recorded the number of rooming-in babies on the unit, the number of rooming-in babies unattended, and the number of unauthorized persons in patient rooms.

3. An assigned staff member stationed at the postpartum nursing unit desk stopped and then recorded every unauthorized person per hour (24 hours a day, 7 days a week).

Control chart data helped to identify a problem with patient education. Some blips were noted on the control chart tracking whether patients were cautioned about leaving their babies unattended. In investigating the blips, staff found that Spanish-speaking patients were not understanding the nurses' cautions. To address the problem, staff produced an information sheet on this and other topics in both Spanish and Arabic—the languages most frequently spoken by the hospital's non-English-speaking patients.

Although initial data indicated some occurrences of unattended babies, there has been only one unattended baby during a 15-month period since January of 1998. Control charts are very effective in letting staff track whether they in fact are reducing the number of unattended babies and unauthorized visitors and holding the gains. Data collection and analysis

Data Collection Tool: Patient Education

Outcome	Yes	No	Comments

1. The mother states her name when the infant is brought to her room.
    Day shift
    Evening shift
    Night shift
	___
	___
	___
		___
		___
		___	

2. The mother is asked to state her ID number at the time the newborn is brought to her room:
    Day shift
    Evening shift
    Night shift
	___
	___
	___
		___
		___
		___	

3. The mother has been told (either by the labor and delivery nurse [L&D] or a Seton 1 nurse) never to leave her infant unattended.			
4. The mother has been told (either by the L&D or a Seton 1 nurse) never to give her infant to an employee who does not have a pink background on the employee ID badge.			

Figure 8-10. This data collection tool was used by nurse managers to capture control chart data on the effectiveness of new mother education. Data collected was used to develop the control charts shown in Figure 8-11, page 184. Tools and instructions were also developed for desk staff and nursing assistants to collect data on visitor access to the unit.
Source: St. Joseph's Hospital and Medical Center, Paterson, NJ. Used with permission.

through control charts has been in place for more than a year and will continue on into the future. Recent control charts for the four measures nurse managers were tracking appear in Figure 8-11, page 184. Staff education efforts continue to be intensive. In January 1999, managers presented the first of what will be annual mandatory in-service education sessions for all staff. Included in the sessions were a review of the hospital's infant safety and security policies and an abductor profile. The staff recently produced a self-learning module, including the hospital's infant identification, infant abduction, and card-receipt policies, with a 20-question posttest to assess competence (see Figure 8-12, page 185). Staff must pass the test with a perfect 100% score in order to work on the unit. Fifty-eight of 59 staff members have passed

the test as of March of 1999. Staff members know that technology-based security improvements are only an adjunct to the education they provide patients and to their continued surveillance on the unit.

Have the improvement initiatives been effective? St. Joseph's Hospital and Medical Center believes that it has clearly demonstrated that each of the recommended remedies definitely has contributed to reducing unauthorized visitors and unattended babies and indeed has been effective. These initiatives and measurements will continue well into the future.

Reference

1. Goodwin TC, Simmons J: Taking charge: Our simple system keeps newborns safe. *RN* 54(5):17–18, 20, 1991.

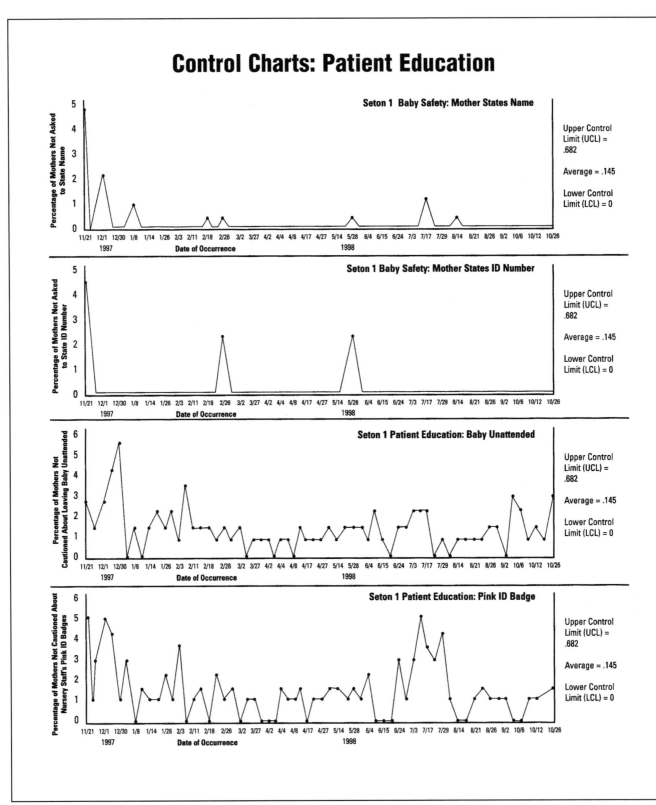

Figure 8-11. These four control charts display the data gathered by nursing managers measuring whether nursing staff asked the mother to state her full name when bringing the baby to her, whether nursing staff asked the mother to read the ID number from her ID band when bringing the baby to her, whether the mother had been cautioned during her stay not to leave her baby unattended, and whether the mother had been cautioned during her stay not to give her baby to anyone without a proper ID badge with a pink background.

Source: St. Joseph's Hospital and Medical Center, Paterson, NJ. Used with permission.

Posttest from Self-Learning Module

St. Joseph's Hospital and Medical Center • Paterson, NJ

Perinatal Unit

Infant Security/Identification Competency

Name: _____   Date of Completion: _____

Score: _____ (Pass or Fail)

Please answer by circling true, false, or the correct letter in the following questions.

T	F	1.	Infant abductors always fit the same description.
T	F	2.	The typical abductor frequently impersonates a hospital staff member.
T	F	3.	The typical abductor is single and living alone.
T	F	4.	The typical abductor is looking for a sibling for another child.
T	F	5.	The typical abductor is emotionally immature and impulsive.
T	F	6.	When an infant is transported for a test, the card receipt goes along with the baby.
T	F	7.	In the event the infant card receipt is lost, a new one gets made out in blue or black ink.
T	F	8.	Infants may be released at the nursery door to anyone who presents the card receipt.
T	F	9.	A hospital staff person may take an infant from the mother's room without the card receipt as long as the hospital staff person has an ID badge with the correct background color.
T	F	10.	On discharge, the mother should be instructed to keep her card receipt.
T	F	11.	When discharging an infant, removal of both ankle ID bands from the baby is acceptable if the mother asks to remove them.
T	F	12.	If the significant other is not present at the delivery, the fourth ID band should be given to the mother so she can give it to that person when he/she comes to visit.
T	F	13.	In the event that an infant's condition is unstable but it has not been determined to which nursery the infant will be admitted, it is acceptable to admit the baby to the regular nursery without a transponder.
T	F	14.	Once the infant and mother are discharged, and the transponder is removed, the mother may walk off the unit as long as there is another person with her.

15. The first action to take in the event of a suspected abduction is
    A. Question the mother regarding the location of the infant
    B. Hold all shifts
    C. Search the unit and do a head count of all babies

16. When an infant is transported between two nurseries, who documents the presence of infant ID bands?
    A. The nurse receiving the baby onto the new unit
    B. The nurse sending (transferring) the baby from the unit
    C. Both A and B

17. Who is responsible for resetting the PROSEC system when it alarms?
    A. Unit clerk
    B. Nurse manager
    C. Nurse in charge during that shift
    D. Security Department staff

18. In the event of a red alarm, what is the first action that should be taken after identifying the location of the alarm?
    A. Call security
    B. Do a head count of all infants if an immediate cause of alarm is not evident
    C. Notify the nurse manager or a 3-11 or 11-7 nurse supervisor

19. Infants receiving tests or x-rays should be transported using which elevator?
    A. "Baby" elevator
    B. Regan elevator
    C. Any elevator is okay to use

20. In the event the ID bands must be corrected, which bands get secured to the infant's chart?
    A. Infant's incorrect band
    B. Mother's incorrect band
    C. Significant other's incorrect band
    D. All of the above

Figure 8-12. This posttest for St. Joseph's self-learning module on infant safety and security must be passed with 100% accuracy for staff to work on Seton 1.

Source: St. Joseph's Hospital and Medical Center, Paterson, NJ. Used with permission.

Glossary of Terms

Accreditation Watch An attribute of an organization's Joint Commission accreditation status. A health care organization is placed on Accreditation Watch when an on-site survey confirms the occurrence of a sentinel event and determines that there is reasonable potential for reducing the likelihood of such events in the future. A health care organization placed on Accreditation Watch is required to execute a thorough and credible root cause analysis. Accreditation Watch status can be publicly disclosed by the Joint Commission.

action plan The product of the root cause analysis that identifies the strategies that an organization intends to implement to reduce the risk of similar events occurring in the future. The plan should address responsibility for implementation, oversight, pilot testing as appropriate, time lines, and strategies for measuring the effectiveness of the actions.

active failure An error that is precipitated by the commission of errors and violations. These are difficult to anticipate and have an immediate adverse affect on safety by breaching, bypassing, or disabling existing defenses.

adverse drug event (adverse drug error) Any incident in which the use of a medication (drug or biologic) at any dose, a medical device, or a special nutritional product (for example, dietary supplement, infant formula, medical food) may have resulted in an adverse outcome in a patient.

adverse event An untoward, undesirable, and usually unanticipated event, such as death of a patient, an employee, or a visitor in a health care organization.

Incidents such as patient falls or improper administration of medications are also considered adverse events, even if there is no permanent effect on the patient.

aggregate To combine standardized data and information.

aggregate data (measurement data) Measurement data collected and reported by organizations as a sum or total over a given time period (for example, monthly, quarterly), or for certain groupings (for example, health care organization level).

aggregate survey data Information on key organization performance areas and standards collected from organizations surveyed by the Joint Commission. This is combined to produce a database of information concerning the performance of the organizations during a specified time interval.

barrier analysis The study of the safeguards that can prevent or mitigate (or could have prevented or mitigated) an unwanted event or occurrence. It offers a structured way to visualize the events related to system failure or the creation of a problem.

benchmarking Continuous measurement of a process, product, or service compared to those of the toughest competitor, to those considered industry leaders, or to similar activities in the organization to find and implement ways to improve it. This is one of the foundations of both total quality management and continuous quality improvement. Internal benchmarking occurs when similar processes within the same organization are compared. Competitive benchmarking occurs when an organization's processes are compared with best practices within the industry. Functional benchmarking refers to benchmarking a similar function or process, such as scheduling, in another industry.

care The provision of accommodations, comfort, and treatment to an individual, implying responsibility for safety, including care, treatment, service, habilitation, rehabilitation, or other programs instituted by the organization for the individual served.

change analysis A study of the differences between the expected and actual performance of a process. Change analysis involves determining the root cause of an event by examining the effects of change and identifying causes.

clinical pathway A treatment regime, agreed on by consensus, that includes all the elements of care, regardless of the effect on patient outcomes. It is a broader look at care and may include tests and X rays that do not affect patient recovery. Synonyms include *clinical path* and *critical pathway*.

common-cause variation *See* variation.

complication A detrimental patient condition that arises during the process of providing health care, regardless of the setting in which the care is provided. For instance, perforation, hemorrhage, bacteremia, and adverse reactions to medication (particularly in the elderly) are four complications of colonoscopy and its associated anesthesia and sedation. A complication may prolong an inpatient's length of stay or lead to other undesirable outcomes.

coupled system A system that links two or more activities so that one process is dependent on another for completion. A system can be loosely or tightly coupled.

error of commission An error that occurs as a result of an action taken. Examples include a drug being administered at the wrong time, in the wrong dose, or using the wrong route; surgeries performed on the wrong side of the body; and transfusion errors involving blood cross-matched for another patient.

error of omission An error that occurs as a result of an action not taken. Examples include a delay in performing an indicated caesarean section, resulting in a fetal death; a nurse omitting a dose of a medication that should be administered; and a patient suicide that is associated with a lapse in carrying out frequent patient checks in a psychiatric unit. Errors of omission may or may not lead to adverse outcomes.

failure Lack of success, nonperformance, nonoccurrence, or the breaking down or ceasing to function. In most instances, and certainly within the context of this book, failure is what is to be avoided. It takes place when a system or part of a system performs in a way that is not intended or desirable.

failure mode and effects analysis (FMEA) A systematic way of examining a design prospectively for possible ways in which failure can occur. It assumes that no matter how knowledgeable or careful people are, errors will occur in some situations and may even be likely to occur. Synonym: *failure mode, effect, and criticality analysis (FMECA)*.

fault tree analysis A systematic way of prospectively examining a design for possible ways in which failure can occur. The analysis considers the possible direct proximate causes that could lead to the event and seeks their origins. Once this is accomplished, ways to avoid these origins and causes must be identified.

flowchart (flow diagram) A pictorial summary that shows with symbols and words the steps, sequence, and relationships of the various operations involved in the performance of a function or a process.

hazard vulnerability analysis The identification of potential emergencies and the direct and indirect effects these emergencies may have on the health care organization's operations and the demand for its services.

hazardous condition Any set of circumstances (exclusive of the disease or condition for which the patient is being treated) which significantly increases the likelihood of a serious adverse outcome. *See also* latent condition.

human factors research The study of the capabilities and limitations of human performance in relation to the design of machines, jobs, and other aspects of the physical environment.

iatrogenic 1. Resulting from the professional activities of physicians, or, more broadly, from the activities of health professionals. 2. Pertaining to an illness or injury resulting from a procedure, therapy, or other element of care.

immediate cause *See* proximate cause.

incident report (occurrence report) A written report, usually completed by a nurse and forwarded to risk management personnel, that describes and provides documentation for any unusual problem, incident, or other situation that is likely to lead to undesirable effects or that varies from established policies and procedures.

indicator 1. A measure used to determine, over time, performance of functions, processes, and outcomes. 2. A statistical value that provides an indication of the condition or direction over time of performance of a defined process or achievement of a defined outcome.

individual served The terms *individual served, patient,* and *care recipient* all describe the individual, client, consumer, or resident who actually receives health care, treatment, and/or service.

Joint Commission International (JCI) JCI extends the Joint Commission's mission worldwide. Through both international consultation and accreditation, JCI helps to improve the quality and safety of patient care in many nations. JCI has extensive international experience working with public and private health care organizations and local governments in more than 40 countries.

Joint Commission on Accreditation of Healthcare Organizations (JCAHO) An independent, not-for-profit organization dedicated to improving the quality of care in organized health care settings. Founded in 1951, its members are the American College of Physicians, the American College of Surgeons, the American Dental Association, the American Hospital Association, and the American Medical Association. The major functions of the Joint Commission include developing accreditation standards, awarding accreditation decisions, and providing education and consultation to health care organizations.

Joint Commission Resources (JCR) A not-for-profit subsidiary of the Joint Commission on Accreditation of Healthcare Organizations, Joint Commission Resources is dedicated to helping health care organizations improve the quality of care and achieve peak performance. JCR offers a full spectrum of resources for health care organizations, including publications, education, consulting and custom education, multimedia products, and the Continuous Survey Readiness initiative, as well as international accreditation and consultation activities. JCR provides expertise on every aspect of accreditation, performance improvement and safety, and other issues health care organizations face today.

latent condition A condition that exists as a consequence of management and organizational processes and poses the greatest danger to complex systems. Latent conditions cannot be foreseen but, if detected, can be corrected before they contribute to mishaps.

licensed independent practitioner (LIP) Any individual permitted by law and by the organization to provide care and services, without direction or supervision, within the scope of the individual's license and consistent with individually granted clinical privileges.

licensed practical nurse (LPN) A nurse who has completed a practical nursing program and is licensed by a state to provide routine patient care under the direction of a registered nurse or a physician. Referred to as *licensed vocational nurse (LVN)* in California and Texas.

licensure A legal right that is granted by a government agency in compliance with a statute governing an occupation (such as medicine or nursing) or the operation of an activity (such as in a long term care facility).

local trigger An intrinsic defect or atypical condition that can create failures.

malpractice Improper or unethical conduct or unreasonable lack of skill by a holder of a professional or official position; often applied to physicians, dentists, lawyers, and public officers to denote negligent or unskillful performance of duties when professional skills are obligatory.

medication Any substance, other than food or devices, that may be used on or administered to persons as an aid in the diagnosis, treatment, or prevention of disease or other abnormal condition. *Synonym:* drug.

medication error A discrepancy between what a physician orders and what is reported to occur. Types of medication errors include omission, unauthorized drug, extra dose, wrong dose, wrong dosage form, wrong rate, deteriorated drug, wrong administration technique, and wrong time. An *omission* medication error is the failure to give an ordered dose; a refused dose is not counted as an error if the nurse responsible for administering the dose tried, but failed, to persuade the patient to take it. Doses withheld according to

written policies, such as for X ray procedures, are not counted as omission errors. An *unauthorized drug* medication error is the administration of a dose of medication not authorized to be given to that patient. Instances of "brand or therapeutic substitution" are counted as unauthorized medication errors only when prohibited by organization policy. A *wrong dose* medication error occurs when a patient receives an amount of medicine that is greater than or less than the amount ordered; the range of allowable deviation is based on each organization's definition. *See also* significant medication errors and significant adverse drug reactions; sentinel event.

near miss Used to describe any process variation that did not affect the outcome, but for which a recurrence carries a significant chance of a serious adverse outcome. Such a near miss falls within the scope of the definition of a sentinel event, but outside the scope of those sentinel events that are subject to review by the Joint Commission under its Sentinel Event Policy.

negligence Failure to use such care as a reasonably prudent and careful person would use under similar circumstances.

observation method An active method of error surveillance in which a trained observer watches the care delivery process.

occurrence report *See* incident report.

occurrence screening A system for concurrent or retrospective identification of adverse patient occurrences (APOs) through medical chart–based review according to objective screening criteria. Examples of criteria include admission for adverse results of outpatient management; readmission for complications; incomplete management of problems on previous hospitalization; or unplanned removal, injury, or repair of an organ or structure during surgery. Criteria are used organizationwide or adapted for departmental or topic-specific screening. Occurrence screening identifies about 80% to 85% of APOs. It will miss APOs that are not identifiable from the medical record.

Official Accreditation Decision Report In the Joint Commission accreditation process, the report resulting from the on-site assessment of an organization or network that outlines identified deficiencies in standards compliance. It also outlines the nature of the accreditation decision, including enumeration of type I recommendations, the remediation of which will be monitored by the Joint Commission through focused surveys or written progress reports. The report may also include other supplemental recommendations that are designed to assist the organization or network in improving its performance.

operative and other procedures Includes operative, other invasive, and noninvasive procedures that place the patient at risk. The focus is on procedures and is not meant to include medications that place the patient at risk.

outcome The result of the performance (or nonperformance) of a function(s) or process(es).

outcome database The database at the Joint Commission that stores the performance measure data and related data elements transmitted by accepted performance measurement systems.

outcome measure A measure that indicates the result of the performance (or nonperformance) of a function(s) or process(es).

Pareto chart A form of vertical bar graph that displays information in such a way that priorities for process improvement can be established. It shows the relative importance of all the data and is used to direct efforts to the largest improvement opportunity by highlighting the "vital few" in contrast to the "many others."

plan-do-study-act (PDSA) cycle A four-part method for discovering and correcting assignable causes to improve the quality of processes. Synonyms: *Deming cycle, Shewhart cycle, plan-do-check-act (PDCA) cycle*.

policies and procedures The formal, approved description of how a governance, management, or clinical care process is defined, organized, and carried out.

practice guidelines Descriptive tools or standardized specification for care of the typical individual in the typical situation, developed through a formal process that incorporates the best scientific evidence of effectiveness with expert opinion. Synonyms include *clinical criteria, parameter* (or *practice parameter*), *protocol, algorithm, review criteria, preferred practice pattern,* and *guideline*.

practice privileges Permission to render care within well-defined limits based on an individual's professional license and his or her training, experience, competence, ability, and judgment.

practitioner Any individual who is qualified to practice a health care profession (for example, a physician or nurse). Practitioners are often required to be licensed as defined by law.

practitioner site The office of a licensed independent practitioner who is a member of the practitioner panel of a PPO or network.

preparedness activities Those activities an organization undertakes to build capacity and identify resources that may be used if an emergency occurs.

prescribing or ordering Directing the selection, preparation, or administration of medication(s).

prevention/early detection (domain) The degree to which appropriate services are provided for promotion, preservation, and restoration of health and early detection of disease.

preventive services Interventions provided by an organization to improve the health status of the populations it serves.

primary source The original source of a specific credential that can verify the accuracy of a qualification reported by an individual health care practitioner. Examples include medical school, graduate medical education program, and state medical board.

privileging The process whereby a specific scope and content of patient care services (that is, clinical privileges) are authorized for a health care practitioner by a health care organization, based on evaluation of the individual's credentials and performance. *See also* licensed independent practitioner (LIP).

procedure 1. A series of steps taken to accomplish a desired end, as in a therapeutic, cosmetic, or surgical procedure. 2. A unit of health care, as in services and procedures.

process A goal-directed, interrelated series of actions, events, mechanisms, or steps that transform inputs into outputs.

proficiency testing 1. The assessment of technical knowledge and skills relating to certain occupations. 2. A peer comparison program used by laboratories to assess reliability of tests performed. Samples, whose precise content is unknown, are provided to laboratories for testing periodically, the results of which are compared with other laboratories that perform the same tests.

proximate cause An act or omission that naturally and directly produces a consequence. It is the superficial or obvious cause for an occurrence. Treating only the "symptoms," or the proximate special cause, may lead to some short-term improvements, but will not prevent the variation from recurring.

public domain (measure) Belonging to the community at large, unprotected by copyright, and subject to

appropriation by anyone.

Public Information Policy A Joint Commission policy governing the confidentiality or disclosure of information about the performance of a health care organization or network. This policy covers the Joint Commission's performance reports, information publicly disclosed on request, complaint information, aggregate performance data, data released to government agencies, and the Joint Commission's right to clarify information an accredited organization releases about its accreditation status.

quality control The performance of processes through which actual performance is measured and compared with goals, and the difference acted upon.

quality improvement An approach to the continuous study and improvement of the processes of providing health care services to meet the needs of individuals and others. Synonyms include *continuous quality improvement, continuous improvement, organizationwide performance improvement,* and *total quality management.*

quality of care The degree to which health services for individuals and populations increase the likelihood of desired health outcomes and are consistent with current professional knowledge. Dimensions of performance include the following: resident perspective issues; safety of the care environment; and accessibility, appropriateness, continuity, effectiveness, efficacy, efficiency, and timeliness of care.

referral The sending of an individual (1) from one clinician to another clinician or specialist, (2) from one setting or service to another, or (3) by one physician (the referring physician) to another physician(s) or other resource, either for consultation or care.

registered nurse (RN) An individual who is qualified by an approved postsecondary program or baccalaureate or higher degree in nursing and licensed by the state, commonwealth, or territory to practice professional nursing.

relevance The applicability and/or pertinence of the indicator to its users and customers. For Joint Commission purposes, face validity is subsumed in this category.

reliability The ability of the indicator to accurately and consistently identify the events it was designed to identify across multiple health care settings.

respect and caring The degree to which those providing services do so with sensitivity for the individual's needs, expectations, and individual differences, and the degree to which the individual or a designee is involved in his or her own care decisions.

restraint Any method (chemical or physical) of restricting a resident's freedom of movement, including seclusion, physical activity, or normal access to his or her body that (1) is not a usual and customary part of a medical diagnostic or treatment procedure to which the resident or his or her legal representative has consented; (2) is not indicated to treat the resident's medical condition or symptoms; or (3) does not promote the resident's independent functioning.

> **chemical restraint** The inappropriate use of a sedating psychotropic drug to manage or control behavior.

> **physical restraint** Any method of physically restricting an individual's freedom of movement, physical activity, or normal access to his or her body. This encompasses many physical devices, such as wrist restraints, jacket vests, and mitts.

risk adjustment A statistical process for reducing, removing, or clarifying the influences of confounding factors that differ among comparison groups (for example, logistic regression, stratification).

risk adjustment data elements Those data elements used to risk adjust a performance measure (such as, reduce, remove, or clarify the influences of confounding resident factors that differ among comparison groups). Such data elements may be used exclusively for risk adjustment (such as not required to construct the numerator or denominator) or may be required for numerator or denominator construction as well as risk adjustment.

risk adjustment model The statistical algorithm that specifies the numerical values and the sequence of calculations used to risk adjust (such as, reduce or remove the influence of confounding factors) performance measures.

risk containment Immediate actions taken to safeguard patients from a repetition of an unwanted occurrence. Actions may involve removing and sequestering drug stocks from pharmacy shelves and checking or replacing oxygen supplies or specific medical devices.

risk management activities Clinical and administrative activities undertaken to identify, evaluate, and reduce the risk of injury to patients, staff, and visitors and the risk of loss to the organization itself.

risk points Specific points in a process that are susceptible to error or system breakdown. They generally result from a flaw in the initial process design, a high degree of dependence on communication, nonstandardized processes, and failure or absence of backup.

root cause The most fundamental reason for the failure or inefficiency of a process.

root cause analysis A process for identifying the basic or causal factor(s) that underlie variation in performance, including the occurrence or possible occurrence of a sentinel event.

safety The degree to which the risk of an intervention (for example, use of a drug or a procedure) and risk in the care environment are reduced for a resident and other persons, including health care practitioners.

safety management A component of an organization's management of the environment of care program that maintains and improves the general safety of the care environment.

scope of care or services The activities performed by governance, managerial, clinical, or support staff.

seclusion Involuntary, solitary confinement of a person where they are physically prevented from leaving the room.

sentinel event An unexpected occurrence involving death or serious physical or psychological injury, or the risk thereof. Serious injury specifically includes loss of limb or function. The phrase *or the risk thereof* includes any process variation for which a recurrence would carry a significant chance of a serious adverse outcome. Such events are called *sentinel* because they signal the need for immediate investigation and response.

> **near miss** Used to describe any process variation that did not affect the outcome, but for which a recurrence carries a significant chance of a serious adverse outcome. Such a near miss falls within the scope of the definition of a sentinel event, but outside the scope of those sentinel events that are subject to review by the Joint Commission under its Sentinel Event Policy.

services Structural divisions of an organization, its medical staff, or its licensed independent practitioner staff; also, the delivery of care.

significant medication errors and significant adverse drug reactions Unintended, undesirable, and unexpected effects of prescribed medications or of medication errors that require discontinuing a medication or modifying the dose; require initial or prolonged hospitalization; result in disability; require treatment with a prescription medication; result in cognitive deterioration or impairment; are life threatening; result in death; or result in congenital anomalies. *See also* medication.

special-cause variation *See* variation.

staff Individuals, such as employees, volunteers, contractors, or temporary agency personnel, who provide services in the organization.

staffing effectiveness The number, competence, and skill mix of staff as related to the provision of needed care, treatment, and service.

staff, medical or licensed independent practitioner Individuals who successfully complete a credentialing process and are granted clinical privileges by the organization.

standard A statement that defines the performance expectations, structures, or processes that must be substantially in place in an organization to enhance the quality of care.

standard deviation A measure of variability that indicates the spread of a set of observations around the mean.

standard of quality A generally accepted, objective standard of measurement, such as a rule or guideline supported through findings from expert consensus, based on specific research and/or documentation in scientific literature against which an individual's or organization's level of performance may be compared.

Statement of Conditions™ (SOC™) A proactive document that helps an organization to do a critical self-assessment of its current level of compliance and describe how to resolve any *Life Safety Code® (LSC®)*

deficiencies. The SOC™ was created to be a "living, ongoing" management tool that should be used in a management process that continually identifies, assesses, and resolves *LSC* deficiencies.

surveillance Ongoing monitoring using methods distinguished by their practicability, uniformity, and rapidity, rather than by complete accuracy. The purpose of surveillance is to detect changes in trend or distribution to initiate investigative or control measures. Active surveillance is systematic and involves review of each case within a defined time frame. Passive surveillance is not systematic. Cases may be reported through written incident reports, verbal accounts, electronic transmission, or telephone hotlines, for example.

surveyor For purposes of Joint Commission accreditation, a physician, nurse, administrator, laboratorian, or any other health care professional who meets the Joint Commission's surveyor selection criteria, evaluates standards compliance, and provides education and consultation regarding standards compliance to surveyed organizations or networks.

survey team The group of health care professionals who work together to perform a Joint Commission accreditation survey.

system database The database at the Joint Commission that stores the profile information for each performance measurement system that has submitted *its* application to the Joint Commission to become a contracted performance measurement system.

tailored survey A Joint Commission survey in which standards from more than one accreditation manual are used in assessing compliance. This type of survey may include using specialist surveyors appropriate to the standards selected for survey.

underlying cause The systems or process cause that allows for the proximate cause of an event to occur. Underlying causes may involve special-cause variation, common-cause variation, or both and may or may not be a root cause.

utilities management A component of an organization's management of the environment of care program designed to ensure the operational reliability, assess the special risks, and respond to failures of utility systems that support the resident care environment.

utility systems Organization systems for life support; surveillance, prevention, and control of infection; environment support; and equipment support. May include electrical distribution; emergency power; vertical and horizontal transport; heating, ventilating, and air conditioning; plumbing, boiler, and steam; piped gases; vacuum systems; or communication systems, including data-exchange systems.

variation The differences in results obtained in measuring the same phenomenon more than once. The sources of variation in a process over time can be grouped into two major classes: common causes and special causes. Excessive variation frequently leads to waste and loss, such as the occurrence of undesirable patient health outcomes and increased cost of health services. **Common-cause variation** (also called *endogenous-cause variation* or *systemic-cause variation*) in a process is due to the process itself and is produced by interactions of variables of that process inherent in all processes, not a disturbance in the process. It can be removed only by making basic changes in the process. **Special-cause variation** (also called *exogenous-cause variation* or *extra-systemic-cause variation*) in performance results from assignable causes. Special-cause variation is intermittent, unpredictable, and unstable. It is not inherently present in a system; rather, it arises from causes that are not part of the system as designed.

Selected Bibliography

Articles

Altman DG: Strategies for community health intervention: Promises, paradoxes, pitfalls. *Psychosom Med* 57(3):226–233, 1995.

Anesthesia Patient Safety Foundation: *APSF Newsletter:* Special issue on office-based anesthesia, Spring 2000.

Barker KN, Allan EL: Research on drug-use-system errors. *Am J Health Syst Pharm* 52(4):400–403, 1995.

Bates DW, et al: Evaluation of screening criteria for adverse events in medical patients. *Med Care* 33(55):452–462, 1995.

Bates DW, et al: Incidence of adverse drug events and potential adverse drug events. Implications for prevention. ADE Prevention Study Group. *JAMA* 274(1):29–34, 1995.

Belkin L: How can we save the next victim? *New York Times Magazine*, Jun 15, 1997, Section 6, pp 28–70.

Berry K, Krizek B: Root cause analysis in response to a "near miss." *J Healthcare Quality* 22: 16–18, Mar/Apr 2000.

Beyea SC, Nicoll LH: When an adverse sentinel event is the cause for action. *AORN Journal* 70: 703–704, Oct 1999.

Blumenthal D: Making medical errors into "medical treasures." *JAMA* 272(23):1867–1868, 1994.

Boyer MM: Root cause analysis in perinatal care: Health care professionals creating safer health care systems. *J Perinatal and Neonatal Nurs* 15: 40–54, May 2001.

Brennan TA, et al: Incidence of adverse events and negligence in hospitalized patients: Results of the Harvard Medical Practice Study I. *N Engl J Med* 324(6):370–376, 1991.

Brennan TA, et al: Identification of adverse events occurring during hospitalization. *Ann Intern Med* 112(3):221–226, 1990.

Campbell GM, Facchinetti NJ: Using process control charts to monitor dispensing and checking errors. *Am J Health Syst Pharm* 55(9):946–954, 1998.

Christensen JF, Levinson W, Dunn PM: The heart of darkness: The impact of perceived mistakes on physicians. *J Gen Intern Med* 7(4):424–431, 1992.

Cohen MR: Drug product characteristics that foster drug-use-system errors. *Am J Health Syst Pharm* 52(4):395–399, 1995.

Colling R: Protect the patients: Hire with care. *Environment of Care News* 1(4):10–11, 1998.

Conley J (ed): RCA 101: Introduction to root cause analysis. *Medical Liability Monitor; Loss Minimizer* supplement, 26(7), Jul 13, 2001.

Cooper JB: Is voluntary reporting of critical events effective for quality assurance? *Anesthesiology* 85(5):961–964, 1996.

Cooper JB, et al: Administrative guidelines for response to an adverse anesthesia event. The Risk Management Committee of the Harvard Medical School's Department of Anaesthesia. *J Clin Anesth* 5(1):79–84, 1993.

Cooper JB, et al: Preventable anesthesia mishaps: A study of human factors. *Anesthesiology* 49(6):399–406, 1978.

Cooper JB, Gaba DM: A strategy for preventing anesthesia accidents. *Int Anesthesiol Clin* 27(3):148–152, 1989.

Cooper JB, Newbower RS, Kitz RJ: An analysis of major errors and equipment failures in anesthesia management: Considerations for prevention and detection. *Anesthesiology* 60(1):34–42, 1984.

Cooper MC: Can a zero defects philosophy be applied to drug errors? *J Adv Nurs* 21(3):487–491, 1995.

Cullen DJ, et al: The incident reporting system does not detect adverse drug events: A problem for quality improvement. *Jt Comm J Qual Improv* 21(10):541–548, 1995.

Dew JR: In search of the root cause. *Qual Prog* 24(3):97–102, 1991.

Feldman SE, Roblin DW: Medical accidents in hospital care: Applications of failure analysis to hospital quality appraisal. *Jt Comm J Qual Improv* 23(11):567–580, 1997.

Ferner RE: Is there a cure for drug errors? *Br Med J* 311(7003):463–464, 1995.

Firestone T: Physical restraints: Meeting the standards/improving the outcomes. *Medsurg Nurs* 7(2):121–123, 1998.

Fleming ST: Complications, adverse events, and iatrogenesis: Classifications and quality of care measurement issues. *Clin Perform Qual Health Care* 4(3):137–147, 1996.

Fletcher CE: Failure mode and effects analysis: An interdisciplinary way to analyze and reduce medication errors. *J Nurs Adm* 27(12):19–26, 1997.

Fox GN: Minimizing prescribing errors in infants and children. *Am Fam Physician* 53(4):1319–1325, 1996.

Gaba DM: Strategies for data collection and analysis to protect patient safety in office-based anesthesia and surgery settings. *Anesthesia Patient Safety Foundation Newsletter* 14, Spring 2000.

Gaba DM: Human error in anesthetic mishaps. *Int Anesthesiol Clin* 27(3):137–147, 1989.

Gaba DM, DeAnda A: The response of anesthesia trainees to simulated critical incidents. *Anesth Analg* 68(4):444–451, 1989.

Gawande A: When doctors make mistakes. *The New Yorker* 74(44):40–55, Feb 1, 1999.

Gobis LJ: Medication errors: Learn from the colleagues' mistakes. *RN* 58(12):59–63, 1995.

Goren S, Abraham I, Doyle N: Reducing violence in a child psychiatric hospital through planned organizational change. *J Child Adolesc Psychiatr Nurs* 9(2):27–28, 37–38, 1996.

Hackel R, Butt L, Banister G: How nurses perceive medication errors. *Nurs Manage* 27(1):31–34, 1996.

Henry T, et al: Learning and process improvement after a sentinel event. *Hosp Pharm* 34(7):839–844, 1999.

Hilfiker D: Facing our mistakes. *N Engl J Med* 310(2):118–122, 1984.

Hirsch KA, Wallace DT: Conduct a cost-effective RCA by brainstorming. *Hospital Peer Review* 24: 105–106, 111–112, Jul 1999.

James BC: Establishing accountability for errors: Who, how, with what impact? Paper presented at the Examining Errors in Health Care Conference, Rancho Mirage, CA: Oct 13–15, 1996.

Joint Commission: *Sentinel Event Alerts* online, Issues 1-27, Feb 1998–June 2002. www.jcaho.org/about+ us/news+letters/sentinel+event+alert/sentinel+event+ alert+index.htm.

Joint Commission: Bedrail-related entrapment deaths. *Sentinel Event Alert*, Issue 27, Sept 6, 2002.

Joint Commission: Delays in treatment. *Sentinel Event Alert*, Issue 26, June 17, 2002.

Joint Commission: Preventing ventilator-related deaths and injuries. *Sentinel Event Alert*, Issue 25, Feb 26, 2002.

Joint Commission: A follow-up review of wrong-site surgery. *Sentinel Event Alert*, Issue 24, Dec 5, 2001.

Joint Commission: Medication errors related to potentially dangerous abbreviations. *Sentinel Event Alert*, Issue 23, Sept 2001.

Joint Commission: Preventing needlestick and sharps injuries. *Sentinel Event Alert*, Issue 22, Aug 2001.

Joint Commission: Medical gas mix-ups. *Sentinel Event Alert*, Issue 21, July 2001.

Joint Commission: Exposure to Creutzfeldt-Jakob Disease. *Sentinel Event Alert*, Issue 20, June 2001.

Joint Commission: Look-alike, sound-alike drug names. *Sentinel Event Alert*, Issue 19, May 2001.

Joint Commission: Kernicterus threatens healthy newborns. *Sentinel Event Alert*, Issue 18, Apr 2001.

Joint Commission: Lessons learned: Fires in the home care setting. *Sentinel Event Alert*, Issue 17, Mar 20, 2001.

Joint Commission: Mix-up leads to a medication error. *Sentinel Event Alert*, Issue 16, Feb 27, 2001.

Joint Commission: Infusion pumps: Preventing future adverse events. *Sentinel Event Alert*, Issue 15, Nov 30, 2000.

Joint Commission: Fatal falls: Lessons for the future. *Sentinel Event Alert*, Issue 14, July 12, 2000.

Joint Commission: Making an impact on health care. *Sentinel Event Alert*, Issue 13, Apr 21, 2000.

Joint Commission: Operative and postoperative complications: Lessons for the future. *Sentinel Event Alert*, Issue 12, Feb 4, 2000.

Joint Commission: High-alert medications and patient safety. *Sentinel Event Alert*, Issue 11, Nov 19, 1999.

Joint Commission: Blood transfusion errors: Preventing future occurrences. *Sentinel Event Alert*, Issue 10, Aug 30, 1999.

Joint Commission: Infant abductions: Preventing future occurrences. *Sentinel Event Alert*, Issue 9, Apr 9, 1999.

Joint Commission: Preventing restraint deaths. *Sentinel Event Alert*, Issue 8, Nov 18, 1998.

Joint Commission: Inpatient suicides: Recommendations for prevention. *Sentinel Event Alert*, Issue 7, Nov 6, 1998.

Joint Commission: Lessons learned: Wrong-site surgery. *Sentinel Event Alert*, Issue 6, Aug 28, 1998.

Joint Commission: Board approves changes to Sentinel Event Policy and Procedures. *Sentinel Event Alert,* Issue 5, July 24, 1998.

Joint Commission: Accreditation committee approves examples of voluntarily reportable Sentinel Events. *Sentinel Event Alert,* Issue 4, May 11, 1998.

Joint Commission: Board approves changes to Sentinel Event Policy and Procedures. *Sentinel Event Alert,* Issue 3, May 1, 1998.

Joint Commission: Board to review modifications to Sentinel Event procedures. *Sentinel Event Alert,* Issue 2, Mar 20, 1998.

Joint Commission: Medication error prevention— Potassium chloride. *Sentinel Event Alert,* Issue 1, Feb 27, 1998.

Kelly WN: Pharmacy contributions to adverse medication events. *Am J Health Syst Pharm* 52(4):385–390, 1995.

Keyes C: Responding to adverse events. *Forum* 18(1):2–3, 1997.

Leape LL: Error in medicine. *JAMA* 272(23):1851–1857, 1994.

Leape LL, et al: Systems analysis of adverse drug events. ADE Prevention Study Group. *JAMA* 274(1):35–43, 1995.

Leape LL, et al: The nature of adverse events in hospitalized patients: Results of the Harvard Medical Practice Study II. *N Engl J Med* 324(6):377–384, 1991.

Lilley LL, Guanci R: Med errors: Applying systems theory. *Am J Nurs* 95(11):14–15, 1995.

Localio AR, et al: Identifying adverse events caused by medical care: Degree of physician agreement in a retrospective chart review. *Ann Intern Med* 125(6):457–464, 1996.

Marek CL: Avoiding prescribing errors: A systematic approach. *J Am Dent Assoc* 127(5):617–623, 1996.

McPhee SJ, et al: Practical issues in disclosing medical mistakes to patients. Presented at the Examining Errors in Health Care Conference, Rancho Mirage, CA: Oct 13–15, 1996.

Mion LD, et al: Physical restraint use in the hospital setting: Unresolved issues and directions for research. *Milbank* Q 74(3):426, 1996.

Moray N: Error reduction as a systems problem. In Bogner MS (ed): *Human Error in Medicine.* Hillsdale, NJ: Lawrence Erlbaum Associates, 1994, pp 70–71.

Nadzam DM: Finding errors before they happen. *Medsurg Nurs* 6(6):370, 1997.

O'Leary DS: Relating autopsy requirements to the contemporary accreditation process. *Arch Pathol Lab Med* 120(8):763–766, 1996.

Pantaleo N, Talan M: Applying the performance improvement team concept to the medication order process. *J Healthc Qual* 20(2):30–35, 1998.

Pepper GA: Errors in drug administration by nurses. *Am J Health Syst Pharm* 52(4):390–395, 1995.

Reason JT: Human and organizational factors: Lessons from other domains. Presented at the Examining Errors in Health Care Conference, Rancho Mirage, CA: Oct 13–15, 1996.

Reichheld FF: Learning from customer defections. *Harv Bus Rev* 74(2):56–69, 1996.

Root cause analysis: Identifying multiple root causes is key to improving performance. *Jt Comm Perspectives on Patient Safety* 2: 4–5, Feb 2002.

Root causes: Improving patient assessment to prevent errors. *Jt Comm Perspectives on Patient Safety* 1: 4-5, Nov 2001.

Root-cause software: Look before you leap. *Hosp Peer Review* 25: 34-5, Mar 2000.

Roseman C, Booker JM: Workload and environmental factors in hospital medication errors. *Nurs Res* 44(4):226–230, 1995.

Rupp RO, Russell JR: The golden rules of process redesign. *Qual Prog* 27(12):85–90, 1994.

Sanborn KV, et al: Detection of intraoperative incidents by electronic scanning of computerized anesthesia records. *Anesthesiology* 85(5):977–987, 1996.

Schwid HA, O'Donnell D: Anesthesiologists' management of simulated critical incidents. *Anesthesiology* 76(4):495–501, 1992.

Senders JW: Detecting, correcting, and interrupting errors. *J Intraven Nurs* 18(1):28–32, 1995.

Shinn JA: Root cause analysis: A method of addressing errors and patient risk. *Prog in Cardiovascular Nurs* 15(1): 24-5, Winter 2000.

Simmons JC: How root-cause analysis can improve patient safety. *The Quality Letter for Healthcare Leaders* 13: 2-12, Oct 2001.

Sluyter GV: Using control charting to address sentinel events and improve organization performance. Presented at the National Conference on Measurement for Improvement in Health Care, Chicago: Nov 11–13, 1998.

Tommasello T: Do substance abuse and dependence contribute to errors in health care? Presented at the Examining Errors in Health Care Conference, Rancho Mirage, CA: Oct 13–15, 1996.

Trick OL: Adverse drug reactions: Establishing a hierarchy of definitions for adjustment of report rates. *Hosp Pharm* 31(12):1593–1595, 1996.

Troutman B, et al: Case study: When restraints are the least restrictive alternative for managing aggression. *J Am Acad Child and Adolesc Psychiatry* 37(5):554–558, 1998.

Turnbull JE, Garrett SE: Hospital develops methods for uncovering underlying causes of error in health care. *QRC Advis* 14(3):1–8, 1998.

Veltman LL: Managing bad results. *Group Practice J* 46(5):26–32, 1997.

Weiss EM: A nationwide pattern of death. *The Hartford Courant*, Oct 11, 1998.

Welch DL: Study of human factors may eliminate errors. *HealthRisk Manag*, 19(9):100–101, 1997.

Willoughby C, Budreau G, Livingston D: A framework for integrated quality improvement. *J Nurs Care Qual* 11(3):44–53, 1997.

Witman AB, Hardin S: Patients' responses to physicians' mistakes. *Forum* 18(4):4–5, 1997.

Wolff AM: Limited adverse occurrence screening: Using medical record review to reduce hospital adverse patient events. *Med J Aust* 164(8):458–461, 1996.

Wu AW et al: To tell the truth: Ethical and practical issues in disclosing medical mistakes to patients. *J Gen Intern Med* 12(12):770–775, 1997.

Zander K: Critical pathways. In Melum MM, Sinioris MK (eds): *Total Quality Management: The Health Care Pioneers.* Chicago: American Hospital Publishing, Inc, 1992, pp 305–314.

Books

Ammerman M: *The Root Cause Analysis Handbook: A Simplified Approach to Identifying, Correcting, and Reporting Workplace Errors*. New York: Quality Resources, 1998.

Andersen B, Fagerhaug T: *Root Cause Analysis: Simplified Tools and Techniques*. Milwaukee, WI: ASQ Quality Press, 2000.

Bogner MS (ed): *Human Error in Medicine*. Hillsdale, NJ: Lawrence Erlbaum Associates, 1994.

Brassard M, Ritter D: *The Memory Jogger™ II*. Methuen, MA: GOAL/QPC, 1994.

Cousins DD (ed): *Medication Use: A Systems Approach to Reducing Errors*. Oakbrook Terrace, IL: Joint Commission Resources, 1998.

Davenport TH: *Process Innovation: Reengineering Work Through Information Technology*. Boston: Harvard Business School Press, 1992.

Gano DL: *Apollo Root Cause Analysis*. Yakima, WA: Apollonian Publications, 1999.

Joint Commission Resources. *Failure Mode and Effects Analysis (FMEA): Proactive Risk Reduction*. Oakbrook Terrace, IL: JCR, 2002.

Joint Commission Resources. *Restraint and Seclusion: Complying with Joint Commission Standards*. Oakbrook Terrace, IL: JCR, 2002.

Joint Commission Resources. *Front Line of Defense: The Role of Nurses in Preventing Sentinel Events*. Oakbrook Terrace, IL: JCR, 2001.

Joint Commission Resources. *Preventing Medication Errors: Strategies for Pharmacies*. Oakbrook Terrace, IL: JCR, 2001.

Joint Commission Resources. *Using Hospital Standards to Prevent Sentinel Events*. Oakbrook Terrace, IL: JCR, 2001.

Joint Commission Resources. *Preventing Patient Suicide*. Oakbrook Terrace, IL: JCR, 2000.

Joint Commission Resources. *Preventing Sentinel Events in the Environment of Care®*. Oakbrook Terrace, IL: JCR, 2000.

Joint Commission Resources. *What Every Hospital Should Know About Sentinel Events*. Oakbrook Terrace, IL: JCR, 2000.

Joint Commission Resources. *Assess for Success: Achieving Excellence with Joint Commission Standards and Baldrige Criteria*. Oakbrook Terrace, IL: JCR, 1999.

Joint Commission Resources. *Preventing Adverse Events in Behavioral Health Care: A Systems Approach to Sentinel Events*. Oakbrook Terrace, IL: JCR, 1999.

Joint Commission Resources. *Medication Use: A Systems Approach to Reducing Errors*. Oakbrook Terrace, IL: JCR, 1998.

Joint Commission Resources. *Reducing Restraint Use in the Acute Care Environment*. Oakbrook Terrace, IL: JCR, 1998.

Joint Commission Resources. *Sentinel Events: Evaluating Cause and Planning Improvement*, 2nd ed. Oakbrook Terrace, IL: JCR, 1998.

Joint Commission Resources. *Storing and Securing Medications*. Oakbrook Terrace, IL: JCR, 1998.

Joint Commission Resources. *Topics in Clinical Care Improvement: Reducing Restraint Use in the Acute Care Environment*. Oakbrook Terrace, IL: JCR, 1998.

Joint Commission Resources. *Topics in Clinical Care Improvement: Storing and Securing Medications*. Oakbrook Terrace, IL: JCR, 1998.

Joint Commission Resources. *A Guide to Performance Improvement in Behavioral Health Care Organizations*. Oakbrook Terrace, IL: JCR, 1996.

Joint Commission Resources. *A Pocket Guide to Using Performance Improvement Tools*. Oakbrook Terrace, IL: JCR, 1996.

Joint Commission Resources. *Using Performance Improvement Tools in Health Care Settings*, Section 6. Oakbrook Terrace, IL: JCR, 1996.

Joint Commission Resources. *Framework for Improving Performance: From Principles to Practice*. Oakbrook Terrace, IL: JCR, 1994.

Juran JM, Gryna FM: Juran's *Quality Control Handbook*, 4th ed. New York: McGraw-Hill, Inc., 1988.

Mobley RK: *Root Cause Failure Analysis*. Boston: Newnes, 1999.

Nelson EC, Batalden PB, Ryer JC (eds): *Clinical Improvement Action Guide*. Oakbrook Terrace, IL: Joint Commission Resources, 1998.

Perrow C: *Normal Accidents: Living with High-Risk Technologies*, 2nd ed. New York: Basic Books, 1999.

Phillips KM: *The Power of Health Care Teams: Strategies for Success*. Oakbrook Terrace, IL: Joint Commission Resources, 1997.

Reason JT: *Managing the Risks of Organizational Accidents*. Brookfield, VT: Ashgate, 1997.

Reason JT: *Human Error*. Cambridge, MA: Cambridge University Press, 1990.

Riegelman RK: *Minimizing Medical Mistakes: The Art of Medical Decision Making*. Boston: Little, Brown and Company, 1991.

Senders JW, Moray NP: *Human Error: Cause, Prediction, and Reduction*. Hillsdale, NJ: Lawrence Erlbaum Associates, 1991.

Sharpe VA: Medical Harm: *Historical, Conceptual, and Ethical Dimensions of Iatrogenic Illness*. Cambridge, MA: Cambridge University Press, 1998.

Index